Praise for The POCU

"... This is the first book of it's kind that has enabled me to reflect on how the politics of prior scientific revolutionaries created the narrative for how I think of POCUS in its current milieu. But Istrail goes a step further and takes a deep dive on the current strength of evidence for the entire body of POCUS only to surface with succinct summaries and useful tables that will convince even the most staunch skeptic. Practically speaking the book is chock full of evidence that those of us on the front lines will deploy when going to battle. I only wish I could have had this perspective 20 years ago when I found myself at the intersection of POCUS naysayers while multiple specialties were warring over who should own this art."

CHRIS FOX MD, CHAIR OF EMERGENCY MEDICINE AND
DIRECTOR OF ULTRASOUND TRAINING, UC IRVINE

"This exemplary book by Dr. Istrail reiterates that for humans, sight serves better than sound."

SANJIV KAUL MD, CHAIR OF CARDIOVASCULAR MEDI-
CINE, OREGON HEALTH & SCIENCE UNIVERSITY, CONTRAST
ECHOCARDIOGRAPHY PIONEER

"When Laennec invented the stethoscope more than 200 years ago, there was a rebellion among doctors to use it. We're seeing a similar unwillingness now for the use of smartphone and pocket ultrasound. In this manifesto, Dr. Istrail makes a solid case for why this technology should reboot the traditional heart and lung physical exam."

ERIC TOPOL MD, ENDOWED CHAIR OF INNOVATIVE
MEDICINE, SCRIPPS RESEARCH, AUTHOR DEEP MEDICINE

"This book is the internal medicine (#IMpocus) clinician's dream. Dr. Istrail beautifully amalgamates the history, medical advances, and techniques of point-of-care ultrasound, and our traditional physical exam with levity and intrigue. It is absolutely fantastic."

RENEE DVERSDAL MD, HOSPITALIST PHYSICIAN,
CHIEF MEDICAL OFFICER OF VAVE HEALTH

"From tamponade to the jugular venous pulse, Dr. Istrail makes a passionate and persuasive case for why point-of-care ultrasound should become the standard of care and bring our bedside exam into the modern era."

HENRY TRAN MD, CARDIOLOGIST, ASSISTANT PROFESSOR
OF MEDICAL EDUCATION, UVA

THE POCUS MANIFESTO

Expanding the limits of our physical exam
with point-of-care ultrasound.

Larry Istrail M.D.

LIBRARY OF CONGRESS CONTROL NUMBER: 2021919198
ISBN: 978-0-578-98009-6 (E-book)
ISBN: 978-0-578-99288-4 (Paperback)

For more information:
www.thepocusmanifesto.com
Twitter: @POCUS_Manifesto
Email: hello@thepocusmanifesto.com

In collaboration with POCUS Med Ed:
www.pocusmeded.com
Twitter: @POCUSMedEd

To my steaming dark roast coffee with a pinch of sugar. You are my rock.

To Max, my first born, my inspiration. Your zeal for food, boundless energy, incessant barking, and cozy furry butt made the pre-dawn writing less lonely.

To my amazing wife who provides unconditional support, and who laughs at my "HOCUS POCUS" jokes every halloween.

And to the woman who collapsed on my flight on the way back from a point-of-care ultrasound conference. Apparently they don't stock ultrasound gel in the medical emergency kits. Fortunately, the glucose gel conducted. Your heart looked great. Glad you were ok.

CONTENTS

INTRODUCTION

For over two centuries of medical history, there has been no more iconic image than the quintessential stethoscope donned confidently over a crisp white coat. This recognizable portrait has been with us in part since 1816, when Dr. Rene Laennec listened through a paper cylinder flush to a patient's chest, revealing a treasure trove of muted thumps, crackles, and wheezes. These sounds and their corresponding causes developed into what we now know as auscultation, the fourth pillar of our physical exam, along with inspection, palpation, and percussion.

Two hundred years later, our treatment options, imaging modalities, and surgical techniques have advanced exponentially while our physical exam, developed at the time of putrid potions and gruesome bloodletting, remains largely unchanged. That is until clinicians began incorporating ultrasound into their patient examination, a practice known as *point-of-care ultrasound*, or **POCUS** for short. POCUS involves using a handheld ultrasound at the bedside to reduce uncertainty, narrow differentials, and guide therapies.

In the eyes of a clinician who has used both a stethoscope and point-of-care ultrasound to examine a patient, the discrepancy in useful information could not prove more stark. In a locked, windowless room, POCUS is the real-time security footage from inside while the stethoscope is an ear and cup flush against the door. POCUS enables a clinician to digitally peel back the skin and observe the ecosystem of internal organs functioning in real-time, an ability our forefathers, foremothers, and stethoscope-monogamous colleagues could infer only through skin changes, audible noises, or subjective symptoms. While ultrasound has been utilized in medicine for decades, POCUS puts this superpower in the hands of the clinician at the bedside to answer clinical questions in real-time, with a tool that is far more accurate than a stethoscope.

With the advent of multiple pocket-sized ultrasound devices propelled by growing clinical evidence at their backs, we are entering a new era in medicine from here on referred to as the *POCUS Era*. The more quickly we accept this reality, the more quickly we can enter an inspiring future of diagnostic medicine and save our patients from preventable complications, near misses, and costly unnecessary tests.

In the relay race of medical progress, the *Before POCUS Era* is nearing the end with its sweat-beaded brow and outstretched arm, ready to pass the baton while POCUS starts its acceleration in the exchange zone. Hippocrates, Laennec, Auenbrugger, Osler, Corvisart, and other medical pioneers have catapulted our physical diagnosis from a palm-reading-equivalent to an empirical assessment. Yet can we not expand upon this foundation two centuries later? Why must we continue to examine our patients in 2021 solely using the techniques of 1821? As the next leg of the race commences, the clinicians unwilling to accept the power and responsibility this baton carries will be left in the dust.

This is not a *how-to* book, but rather a *why* book. In what follows, basic stethoscopic and sonographic concepts and the evidence to support them will be presented through the lens of the relevant medical history on which our current medical diagnostic knowledge resides. While some clinicians are now familiar with the concept of POCUS, this book additionally hopes to target the many other physicians, medical students, nurse practitioners, physician assistants, paramedics, or anyone else who uses a stethoscope that may not fully appreciate the potential POCUS offers. While point-of-care ultrasound can be used to examine almost any part of the body, this book focuses exclusively on diseases of the thorax.

What POCUS *isn't* is a replacement for standard imaging or physical examination. Traditional echocardiograms, CT scans, and MRIs, venous and arterial doppler exams often (but not always) provide much more detailed information than POCUS should or could. Rather, POCUS is an inspector-gadget-like augmentation of our physical exam: examine the patient's skin, muscle tone, reflexes, and heart sounds, but also sonographically inspect the internal jugular vein, the carotid artery, chambers of the heart, and the lungs.

Part I examines our abilities to diagnose diseases of the lungs. It begins with the origins of the stethoscope and our physical exam techniques dating back to the 1700s, as well as the evidence to support such methods. This is followed by the early days of lung ultrasound, how it has evolved, and how the evidence compares to that of auscultation in the diagnosis of pulmonary disease. Part II discusses cardiovascular disease, and how the stethoscope and focused cardiac ultrasound compare in their diagnostic capabilities. Finally, Part III discusses criticisms and praise evoked against, or in defense of, incorporating POCUS into our standard physical exam.

PART I

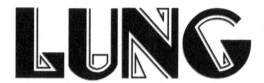

"In the history of mankind, it will be found, that no great discovery, or probably conjecture was ever promulgated, without encountering the most bitter opposition. Harvey was thought a dreamer, yet he proved the circulation of the blood; and Columbus was laughed at as a projector, until he returned with the spoils of the west. But in this enlightened age, let us not judge with our eyes shut. Mediate auscultation, like truth, does not shrink from inquiry, but, on the contrary, courts investigation. Her advocates only demand a fair trial; they enter the lists with confidence, and bear for their motto the saying of the wise man, "That a new fact is a new friend; and when we have gotten rid of an error, we have, in reality, conquered an enemy."

DR. WILLIAM STOKES, 1825

An Introduction to the Use of the Stethoscope

CHAPTER 1: PHYSICAL EXAM ORIGINS

"When ... we hear ... that certain persons have tried the stethoscope, and abandoned it upon finding it useless or deceptive; and when we learn, on inquiry, that the trial was extended merely to the hurried examination of a few cases ... we can only regret that such students should have been so misdirected, or should have so misunderstood the fundamental principles of the method. No conclusions, deduced from such attempts - I cannot dignify them with the term 'experience' - can have any weight with those qualified to judge the matter."

DR. JOHN FORBES, 1830

The thorax is truly one of life's miracles. If devised on a 3-D printer today it would be difficult to improve upon the elegant design awarded to us in utero. A hard, bony cage made up of rounded, cylindrical ribs that sinusoidally project from the vertebrae to the sternum. Sitting inside this protective enclosure are two organs that, when healthy, are most responsible for maintaining life, yet when diseased, most culpable for squandering it. "It may even be asserted, that in maladies of every sort, whatever be their seat, death scarcely ever occurs without the chest becoming affected in one way or other," described medical pioneer and inventor of the stethoscope Dr. Rene Laennec, "and that, in most cases, life does not seem in peril until ... a congested state of the lungs, serous effusion in the pleura, or great disorder of the circulation."[1]

Until the 1760s, the thorax was analogous to an airplane's black box: unassuming during life, yet essential to understanding what went wrong after death. While the post mortem anatomy had been worked out by the likes of Andreas Vesalius in the 1500s and Giovanni Battista Morgagni in the 1700s, understanding how organs fail and how to diagnose their failures in alive humans was still largely a mystery.[2]

Leopold Auenbrugger, born in 1722, was an Innkeeper's son and one of the first to try to unpack this puzzle (Figure 1). He became a physician in the Spanish Military Hospital in Vienna, Austria, and discovered that tapping the chest in ill patients yielded different sounds in different locations. He developed this observation into a method of disease localization and assessment of the organs within. He called it *percussion* and honed his craft by comparing his findings with post mortem dissections, notably filling cadaver chests with water to determine how fluid alters the percussion's sound. As the story goes, his epiphany to use percussion came from seeing his father working at the Inn, tapping wine barrels to determine the fluid level inside.[3] Auenbrugger was also likely influenced by his musical background, even writing the libretto of an opera that was performed repeatedly in Vienna during that time.[4]

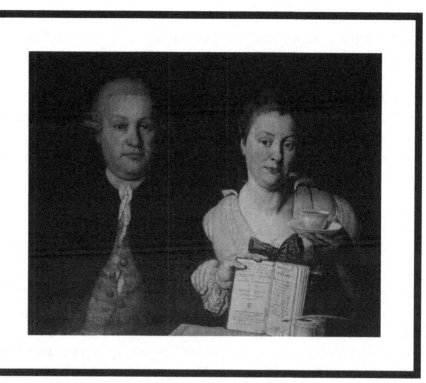

FIGURE 1   Dr. Leopold Auenbrugger (1722 - 1809) who first developed the method of Percussion. Pictured here with his wife.

Public Domain image from Wikipedia.
Via https://bit.ly/3F9nRWH

He published *New Invention by Means of Percussing the Human Thorax for Detecting Signs of Obscure Disease of the Interior of the Chest* in 1761, describing this new technique:

> *"I here present the reader with a new sign which I have discovered for detecting diseases of the chest. This consists in percussion of the human thorax, whereby, according to the character of the particular sounds thence elicited, an opinion is formed of the internal state of that cavity."*

Auenbrugger recommended percussion be done with a hand gloved in unpolished leather, or that the patient's chest be covered in a tight-fitting shirt. A normal sound "resembles the stifled sound of a drum covered with a thick woolen cloth," he explained, compared to a region of the chest that is "entirely destitute of the natural sounds - that is, if it yields only a sound like that of a fleshy limb when struck—disease exists in that region."[2]

He eventually settled upon four percussion notes: normal, tympanitic, dullness, and flatness, and mapped them to various disease states, comprising the first systematic method of decoding the mysteries inside the living thorax. However, his work went largely unnoticed for almost 50 years until it was discovered by Dr. Jean Nicolas Corvisart, one of France's great physicians at the time. With the claim to fame of being Napoleon Bonepart's personal doctor, Corvisart was well respected and began using percussion in his own practice. He eventually published a French translation of Auenbrugger's text with his own additions in 1808, just one year before Auenbrugger's death.[5]

With Corvisart's influence, this technique gained popularity in Paris and seemed to become the standard of care. As one physician reported in 1820, "a patient brought to any of the hospitals in Paris with any affection of the chest, is as regularly submitted to [percussion] as the English physician would ascertain the state of the pulse."[5] This excitement was short-lived however, as just eight years after Corvisart's publication, a new tool was invented that would forever change how patients are examined. "[P]ercussion, it is true, was had recourse to, but only in latter times has this method been brought to the scanty perfection of which it is capable," wrote famed Irish physician Dr. William Stokes in his 1825 text An Introduction to the Use of the Stethoscope.[6] "Percussion alone is in many cases useless, but as, when combined with mediate auscultation, it becomes of the highest value."

Auenbrugger's work was a profound first step in the development of the modern physical exam, yet went largely ignored for most of his life. Fortunately, Corvisart's clout helped spread it into the medical community, and into the hands of one man in particular.

CHAPTER 2: THE STETHOSCOPE & MEDIATE AUSCULTATION

"It must be confessed that there is something even ludicrous in the picture of a grave physician formally listening through a long tube applied to the patient's thorax, as if the disease within were a living being that could communicate its condition to the sense without."

DR. JOHN FORBES, 1821

The word *stethoscope* comes from *Stetho* in ancient Greek which translates to 'chest,' and *Skopeo*, which is 'to examine, inspect, or look into.' It was coined by one of medicine's great pioneers, a young French physician named Rene Theophile Hyacinthe Laennec. Born in Quimper in the northwest portion of France in 1781, he had a difficult childhood characterized by frequent illness and hardship. At five years of age, his mother died of tuberculosis,[1] and at 12 he moved to Nantes to live with his uncle Guillaume François Laennec, a physician and dean of the faculty of medicine at the university there. Inspired by his uncle's work, Laennec cared for the sick and wounded of the French Revolution at Hôtel Dieu in Nantes, and by 18 was working in the Military hospital.[7] In 1800, he traveled to Paris to complete his medical education at a clinical school by the name of *École Pratique,* learning from many famed scientists and physicians, most notably Napoléon Bonaparte's very own Dr. Jean Corvisart.

Laennec was an extremely motivated medical student, publishing his first papers on topics such as peritonitis, amenorrhea, and liver disease, while also serving as the editor of a medical journal. He quickly became distinguished amongst his peers, in no small part to the fact that during his first three years in medical school, he "drew up a minute history of nearly four hundred cases of disease,"[1] many of which would later become the fodder for his famous text.

He continued his industrious nature as a physician after graduating medical school and in 1816 was appointed chief physician to Necker Hospital in Paris. It was here where he spent years characterizing various diseases through correlation of clinical and post mortem exams. This knowledge culminated in his seminal textbook, *A Treatise on the Diseases of the Chest and on Mediate Auscultation,* initially published in 1819 and translated to English shortly after.[8]

It was under the famed Dr. Corvisart where he first learned about Auenbrugger's percussion method. Laennec felt it was "one of the most valuable discoveries ever made in medicine. By means of it, several diseases which had hitherto been cognisable by general and equivocal signs only, are brought within the immediate sphere of our perceptions, and their diagnosis, consequently, rendered both easy and certain."[1] Yet it left him with much to be desired, as percussion as a diagnostic tool "was very incomplete," and was "confined, in a great measure, to the indication of fullness or emptiness, it is only applicable to a limited number of organic lesions."

Immediate auscultation, or placing the ear directly on the chest, was another technique dating back to Hippocrates.[9] This theoretically offered more information than percussion could, however, according to Dr. Stokes was "far from giving the satisfactory results which it would seem to promise. The sounds which are thus heard are not perfectly distinct ... transmitted by the whole surface of the head, which is in contact with the chest, they appear to have so much intensity that we cannot appreciate their shades of difference." It is also understandably uncomfortable, as the ear "cannot be placed on every point of the thorax, particularly among females, where decency alone suffices to interdict this mode of auscultation."[6]

In fact, it was this desire for decency, at least in part, that sparked Laennec's idea to create the stethoscope. As he explained his revelation in 1816:[1]

> "I was consulted by a young woman laboring under general symptoms of diseased heart, and in whose case percussion and the application of the hand were of little avail on account of the great degree of fatness. The other method just mentioned [that is, immediate auscultation] being rendered inadmissible by the age and sex of the patient, I happened to recollect a simple and well-known fact in acoustics, and fancied, at the same time, that it might be turned to some use on the present occasion. The fact I allude to is the augmented impression of sound when conveyed through certain solid bodies - as when we hear the scratch of a pin at one end of a piece of wood, on applying our ear to the other. Immediately, on this suggestion, I rolled a quire of paper into a kind of cylinder and applied one end of it to the region of the heart and the other to my ear, and was not a little surprised and pleased, to find that I could thereby perceive the action of the heart in a manner much more clear and distinct than I had ever been able to do by the immediate application of the ear."

This **mediate auscultation** through a stethoscope was more precise and offered patients more modesty during their clinical exam, providing a focal, audible window into the chest of a living person (Figure 2). It was a new diagnostic technique that offered "a set of new signs ... to render the diagnosis of diseases of the lungs, heart and pleura," creating what we now know as the field of auscultation, the fourth pillar of our modern-day physical exam, along with inspection, palpation, and percussion.

It also provided Laennec with an awesome vision of what the physical exam could become. "From this moment I imagined that the circumstance might furnish means for enabling us to ascertain the character, not only of the action of the heart, but of every species of sound produced by the motion of all the thoracic viscera, and, consequently, for the exploration of the respiration, the voice, the rattle or rhonchus, and perhaps even the fluctuation of fluid extravasated in the pleura or the pericardium."

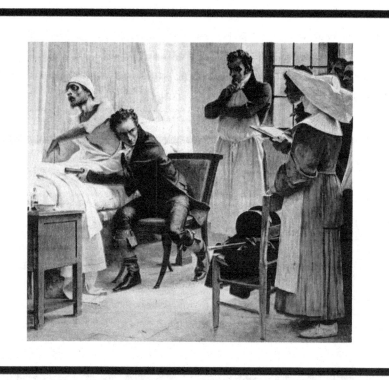

FIGURE 2 Dr. Rene Laennec (1781 - 1826) using his stethoscope to examine a patient in front of students at Necker Hospital.

Public Domain image from Wikipedia.
Painting by Théobald Chartran
https://bit.ly/3kUb3vb

The living thorax was a medical mystery and Laennec's stethoscope was one of the first decryption devices. Initially constructed of "three quires of paper, compactly rolled into a cylinder and kept in that shape by means of paste," it eventually morphed into a hollow walnut structure that improved the usability and acoustics.[10] A device, he noted, that could only be validated in a hospital setting which allowed the possibility to verify "by examination after death, the diagnostics established by means of the cylinder." It was this validation through examining nearly 3,000 patients[11] that culminated in Laennec's life's work. Less than two years after his discovery, he read a memoir before the Academy of Sciences containing the outlines of his new method, and one year later, in 1819 he published his immortal work in his native French language. It was translated into English by a Scottish physician named Sir John Forbes, and on August 13th, 1824, London's *Morning Chronicle* announced its publication (Figure 3).[12]

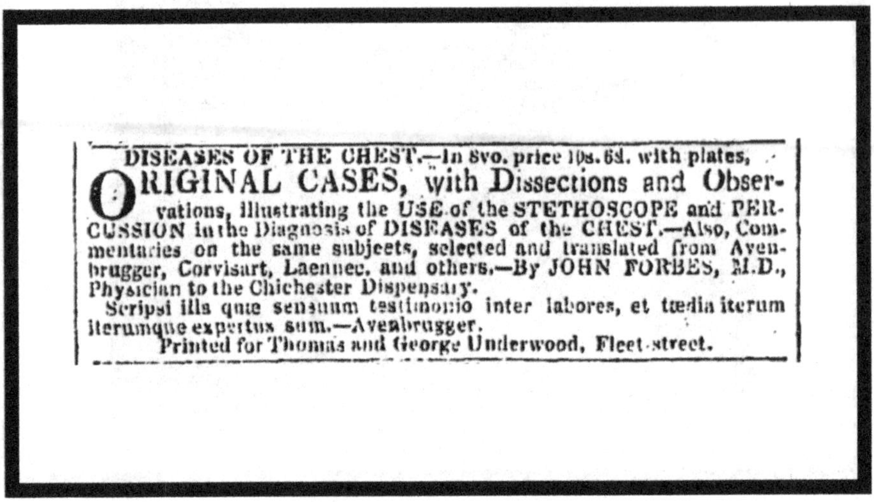

DISEASES OF THE CHEST.—In 8vo. price 10s.6d. with plates,

ORIGINAL CASES, with Dissections and Observations, illustrating the USE of the STETHOSCOPE and PERCUSSION in the Diagnosis of DISEASES of the CHEST.—Also, Commentaries on the same subjects, selected and translated from Avenbrugger, Corvisart, Laennec, and others.—By JOHN FORBES, M.D., Physician to the Chichester Dispensary.

Scripsi illa quæ sensuum testimonio inter labores, et tædia iterum iterumque expertus sum.—Avenbrugger.

Printed for Thomas and George Underwood, Fleet-street.

FIGURE 3 Original newspaper announcement for the publication of the English translation of Dr. Laennec's *Treatise on Diseases of the Chest and on Mediate Auscultation*. London Morning Chronicle, August 13th, 1824.

London Morning Chronicle Archive
Via newspapers.com

Stethoscope Meets Resistance

Laennec's new book introduced the world to his cylindrical device and a new field of mediate auscultation to accompany it. Like any new technology however, the stethoscope was initially received with considerable skepticism. "Although it has a very fine name, it is, after all, nothing more than a stick with a hole in it" wrote one lawyer in an 1835 lawsuit.[13] Francois Broussais, a French physician at the time was a fierce critic of Laennec and the stethoscope, accusing him of plagiarism, and labeled his text as "obscure ... sad, and cluttered with a mass of meaningless facts and useless peculiarities."[11] Other physicians felt using a stethoscope "leads to no practical results, and therefore that it is more useful to the pathologist than the physician."[6]

Yet stethoscopy as it was called, attracted many supporters from around Europe who traveled to Paris, eager to learn from Laennec. At a time with no internet or global book distribution, the adoption of this new technique was largely influenced by just a few individual physicians. One was Dr. John Forbes, who enabled broader awareness by translating Lannec's text into English. Another was Dr. William Stokes, an Irish physician most famous for lending his name to 'Cheyne-Stokes breathing.' He was a professor of medicine at the University of Dublin and an early believer in what the stethoscope could offer. In fact, he was so impressed by this new device that he wrote his own book on the stethoscope written in English and published in 1825, summarizing much of Laennec's work into a more practical guide. He felt strongly that those who objected to the use of this device "like unjust judges, pronounce sentence without examining the merits of the case."[6]

The technique spread throughout England, where "[t]he stethoscope was laughed at, in the first instance, by the English," but slowly gained acceptance as more people saw it being used, convincing "many persons of the importance of this instrument" wrote a physician named Francis Cox in the Derby Mercury newspaper in 1830.[14] It gained enough momentum to the point that within a decade, some physicians felt that not using a stethoscope to examine their patients would jeopardize their reputation.[2] However, this was not the position held by all doctors. "Few intelligent physicians ... refuse to acknowledge that the discovery of Laennec forms a memorable epoch in the history of medicine," wrote Dr. Austin Flint, an influential physician from the late 1850s, yet "the number who give much attention to the principles and practice of physical exploration is quite small, its advantages being practically rejected by a large proportion of the medical profession."[15]

The late 19th and early 20th century saw many advances to the stethoscope to improve its form and function. The two earpieces were added by George Philip Cammann in the 1850s. This design lasted about 100 years, until Dr. David Littmann, a cardiologist at Harvard Medical School created a newer version that was lighter and had better acoustics. His business *Cardiosonics, Inc* was acquired by a bigger company named *3M* that has since become one of the main manufacturers and distributors of stethoscopes worldwide, bearing Dr. Littmann's surname on each one.[16]

The stethoscope evolved from a rolled-up paper cylinder into a rubber tubed listening device optimized to pick up cardiopulmonary sounds. To this day it still relies on the principles Laennec first described 200 years ago: that a diseased organ emits an SOS signal in its native tongue of wheezes and rales, and it is the clinician's job, with the help of a stethoscope, to translate these sounds into actionable diagnoses. This is the foundation by which our modern clinical exam resides, a tribute to Laennec and his meticulous life's work.

CHAPTER 3: LUNG AUSCULTATION

The heart and lungs comprise the two working units of the cardiopulmonary system. The heart is made up of two connected pumps: the **left heart**, which pumps oxygenated blood to the body, and the **right heart**, which pumps deoxygenated blood to the lungs. The left and right hearts are connected like two merging interstate highways, with the blood being shuttled through an ever-shrinking conduit system from a roughly 3-cm diameter aorta down to an 8-micron capillary just larger than a single red blood cell.[17] This system allows for a streamlined recirculation of blood around your body, but it can lead to trouble when one of the pumps isn't working properly.

If the **left ventricle** is damaged and only works at 50% capacity for example, then fluid will congest upstream into the lungs and cause shortness of breath. "The blood, not being freely transmitted by the left ventricle," as 19th-century cardiologist Dr. James Hope described it in 1839, "accumulates in the lungs," and propagates this engorgement "backwards to the right side of the heart, to the great veins, and finally to all their ramifications."[18] This **congestive heart failure** as we now know it, is one of the most common causes of hospitalization in the United States each year.[19] In these patients, the shortness of breath is largely caused by pulmonary edema which "is rarely a primary and idiopathic disease," Laennec explained, rather "comes on, most commonly, with other dropsical [that is, those that cause swelling] affections ... especially those of the heart."[1]

When examining a patient with edema of the lungs, Laennec described "a slight crepitation" when listening through a stethoscope, "as in the degree of peripneumony, more like a rattle than the natural sounds of respiration." He detailed this in a case of a 47-year-old woman that later succumbed to the condition:

> "She came into the Hospital a fortnight thereafter [her symptoms started], affected with edema of the superior extremities, particularly the left - dyspnea and cough, with expectoration of white viscid sputua ... the anasarca [i.e. swelling] greatly increased, and extended over the whole body, except the face ... it was found, on applying the stethoscope, that the respiration was very distinct on both sides anteriorly, and was accompanied by a slight crepitous rattle on the lower parts of the sides and back. She died about three months after her admission."

Thirty hours after her death, Laennec performed an autopsy and found that the tissue corresponding to the area where he heard those rattling breath sounds "contained somewhat less than a pint of limpid serum," but otherwise looked normal, "of a pale rose-colour, free from tubercles and exhibiting no trace of peripneumony, nor even sanguinous congestion." Laennec was describing what he called **rales,** also known today as pulmonary **crackles.** He thought they sounded like "the fine crackling of roasting fat," or the "crackling of salt on hot coals," and that "with very few exceptions, they indicate the presence of liquids in the bronchial tubes."

Characterizing Lung Sounds

In experimenting with his new tool, Laennec was struck by a revelation when evaluating a woman "with a slight bilious fever, and a recent cough having the character of a pulmonary catarrh." When he placed the stethoscope below the right clavicle, "her voice seemed to come directly from the chest, and to reach the ear through the central canal of the instrument," a bizarre phenomenon that was only present in one square inch of her lung. He detected these sounds in patients with advanced tuberculosis as well, calling it **pectoriloquism,** and correctly concluding it was due to areas of the lung where "tuberculous excavations" were present.[2]

With each pulmonary disease, from pulmonary hemorrhage to cancer, asthma to effusions, he documented his experience with each one in stunning detail. Through his careful assessment of hundreds of lungs, he came across nonspecific but abnormal sounds he termed **rattles** or **rhonchi** to "express all the sounds, beside those of health, which the act of respiration gives rise to." There was the **dry sonorous rhonchus,** which resembled "the snoring of a person asleep ... and occasionally the cooing of the wood pigeon." In fact, in some patients, he felt this sound was so similar to a bird's squawk "that we might be tempted to believe the bird concealed under the patient's bed." Also notable was the **dry sibilous rattle** which sounded like "the chirping of birds, the sound emitted by suddenly separating two portions of smooth oiled stone, or by the action of a small valve." Patient after patient, Laennec developed a catalog of "rales, and hissing, whistling, and sonorous sounds" heard through auscultation and what post mortem findings they corresponded to.

Pneumothorax, Pleural Effusions & Empyema

In his autopsies of patients with shortness of breath or cough, Laennec commonly saw fluid or air encased in the chest cavity, outside the lungs. These findings were named in reference to the type of fluid present, whether "of pus, of blood, of water and air are often used synonyms of pleurisy, hemothorax, hydrothorax, and pneumothorax." In order to differentiate the type of effusion when the patient was still alive, his auscultation and percussion abilities were often not sufficient, and he relied on the teachings of Hippocrates and a method called *succussion*. "If auscultation by itself cannot, as Hippocrates supposed, detect the presence of a fluid in the chest, we obtain, at least, from the writings of this great man ... a sign very characteristic of this affection, in one particular form of it. This method of exploration ... consists of shaking the patient's trunk, and at the same time listening to the sounds thereby produced." Hippocrates explained that in patients with pus in their thoracic cavity, there is viscous infectious fluid present and therefore "those who produce most sound when shaken by the shoulder, have less pus in the chest than those who yield less sound," and that those who do not produce any sounds during this technique "are full of pus and their case is desperate." In the case of pneumothorax, Laennec could adeptly arrive at the correct diagnosis with his stethoscope and percussion alone, noting that if one side of the chest had distinct breath sounds while "not at all on the other, - we may be assured that there exists a pneumothorax on the latter."

While Laennec is most well known for his development of the stethoscope, almost equally noteworthy was his work ethic and dedication to the field of medicine. Without the benefit of EKGs, radiology, pulse oximeters, or modern medical knowledge, Laennec was able to advance our understanding of cardiac and pulmonary disease while developing a new field of diagnostic medicine in the process. However, what he did not explore was how common these characteristic sounds are in the general population. Do these lung crackles and wheezes exist in healthy patients as well? Or on the contrary, how commonly does cardiopulmonary disease manifest inaudibly to the human ear? The answers to these questions lie in the sensitivity and specificity of his exam findings, the key to understanding how accurate they actually were.

CHAPTER 4: DIAGNOSIS & SCREENING WITH AUSCULTATION

"Such are the different affections of the chest, which, in this point of view, are perhaps of more importance than those of any other cavity in the human body. Before the discovery of auscultation, the diagnosis of these affections was obscure and difficult; many and fatal must have been the errors into which medical men fell in the absence of such a light."

DR. WILLIAM STOKES, 1825

The teachings of Auenbrugger, Laennec, Stokes, Osler, Corvisart, and many others have been ceremonially passed to each new generation of doctors in the tradition-preserving, right of passage teachings at the bedside. Classically this consists of an attending physician listening as the medical case is presented by a medical student or clinician-in-training. This medical team then evaluates the patient together, learning from the attending as they examine the patient and offer wisdom to their trainees. This is a tradition that has continued since the late 1800s, however, like an inter-generational game of telephone, our proficiency has progressively waned. This decline in clinical acumen is evidenced by medical trainees' poor performance with basic physical exam skills.[20] While there are many reasons for this devolution of expertise, one is certainly the increasing reliance on CT scans, echocardiograms, and other advanced imaging techniques.

While it is unfortunate, to some degree it is also expected. An experienced taxi cab driver who knows every coffee shop and back road in town once offered tremendous benefit to those looking to get through a city efficiently. However, with the advent of Google Maps, even the most experienced driver cannot compete with real-time traffic data and calculated routes. This creates a strong disincentive for young new drivers to develop or maintain a cognitive map of a given city when it can be accomplished far quicker and more accurately with a smartphone.

Likewise, watching a physician who trained in the time before advanced imaging is like watching a brilliant detective at a crime scene. Finding clues in seemingly unrelated places: nail bed black streaks (i.e. *splinter hemorrhages*) to diagnose an infected heart valve, for example. Like *Sherlock Holmes*, such clinicians make medicine inspiring and interesting. For every correct diagnosis though, how many are missed due to poor sensitivity of a given exam finding? Exploring the diagnostic accuracy of auscultation offers some insight into this question.

We should first understand that while certain auscultated or physical exam findings are *associated* with various diseases, they are not necessarily sensitive or specific for that disease. Are lung crackles detected in 100% of patients with pulmonary edema? Or is it closer to 10%? Along the same lines, when crackles *are* heard, does that mean pulmonary edema exists 100% of the time?

Kidneys, Lobsters & Lung Rales

An ideal screening or diagnostic exam has multiple criteria that need to be met. Arguably the most important is high accuracy,[21] the key to which is its sensitivity and specificity. A flawless screening test or physical examination would have 100% sensitivity and 100% specificity, meaning every case was detected without any false positives or false negatives. In reality however, tests are rarely this precise.

It is worth better understanding these terms before moving on.

Suppose there is a lobster fisherman named Gunther. Gunther is looking to increase his lobster yield with each outing in a part of the ocean with 100 lobsters and 100 tuna fish. His current lobster cage is a rusty wire box that is submerged into the ocean, catching 70 lobsters and 30 tuna fish each time. Thirty lobsters are left in the sea and he cannot sell the tuna fish. This cage is therefore 70% sensitive for lobster. Since it also catches tuna fish, it is not very specific to lobsters either. Gunther devises a new lobster trap with lobster bait and tuna fish repellent, allowing him to catch all the lobsters and only the lobsters. This would be 100% sensitive and 100% specific to the lobsters in that ocean.

This same framework should be applied to our physical exam. When evaluating a patient with shortness of breath, for example, is lung auscultation the upgraded lobster catcher or the rusty box? Or is it even worse?

Italian researchers in 2016 sought to answer this question, studying the ability of lung auscultation to detect pulmonary edema. They studied patients with end-stage renal disease, due to the fact that a patient right before dialysis with shortness of breath will have a lot of pulmonary edema, most of which will be removed after dialysis. They performed over 1,000 exams on 79 patients before and after dialysis for over a year, listening to their lungs for crackles and examining their extremities for soft tissue swelling. What they found was not flattering to the *Before*

POCUS Era.

Lung crackles were not present in 61% of patients with moderate to severe pulmonary edema, and in patients with severe lung congestion, crackles were only present half the time. Even more disheartening was the fact that peripheral edema was conspicuously absent over 80% of the time in patients with moderate to severe pulmonary edema, computing a false negative rate of over 70%.[22] This study "shows that the two time-honored clinical signs, like lung crackles and peripheral edema, that are universally applied to detect and monitor volume excess ... have an unsuspectedly low sensitivity for detecting interstitial edema in a most critical organ, like the lungs," and that "these clinical signs only remotely reflect the degree of lung congestion."

These results suggest that the ways we typically assess patients with suspected pulmonary edema cannot effectively detect it. Similarly, in another study of 250 emergency room patients who presented with shortness of breath, rales were only 56% sensitive and 80% specific for detecting pulmonary edema,[23] while in a study of ICU patients, lung auscultation was only 34% sensitive for detecting it.[24]

In other conditions that cause lung crackles like interstitial lung disease, physicians were only able to pick up about six out of ten cases with auscultation alone.[25] To complicate matters further, the prevalence of lung crackles increases as we age, to the point where up to 70% of asymptomatic patients over 80 may have lung crackles without known pulmonary disease. And in younger adults, crackles can be heard more than 30% of the time in otherwise normal lungs confirmed on high-resolution CT scans.[26]

Ultimately the question comes down to this: *how effective is the stethoscope to detect and assess pulmonary disease, and compared to what?* Compared to not listening at all it seems to provide benefits, but just how much does it improve our clinical assessment?

Researchers in the Netherlands performed a meta-analysis to determine if the stethoscope, "200 years after its invention [is] ready to be relegated to the museum shelf or does [it] still provide vital clues to aid in the diagnosis?" In 2020, they published their results in *Nature* including thirty-four studies that examined lung auscultation accuracy in four common lung diseases: congestive heart failure, asthma, chronic obstructive pulmonary disease (COPD), and pneumothorax. Combining all diseases they found an overall pooled sensitivity of 37%.[27] Out of 100 lobsters, this net only caught 37.

The absence of breath sounds had very good diagnostic accuracy for picking up a pneumothorax, hemothorax, or pleural effusion, but could not differentiate between them. Lung crackles were only 64% sensitive and 66% specific for detecting congestive heart failure related pulmonary crackles, and the presence or absence of crackles "only marginally alter[ed] the provisional diagnosis." For asthma or COPD, wheezing was quite specific at 93% but only 25% sensitive, and for pneumonia, the accuracy was quite poor as well. The authors concluded that lung auscultation is "not clinically useful in making a diagnosis in most circumstances," and that "we must reconsider the use of the stethoscope in patient groups with low prevalence of disease and in clinical situations where more advanced diagnostic modalities are available. Only in clinical situations in resource limited areas, with high prevalence of disease and in experienced hands the stethoscope has some clinical relevance."

A Bitter Pill for the *Before POCUS Era*

The stethoscope is the doctor's defining icon, the final accessory to complete the professional look, a tacit demand of respect from trainees and patients alike. Yet it is not without its flaws.

The diagnostic accuracy of auscultation for lung pathologies is consistently poor, and its primary role in assessing pulmonary disease should be reconsidered now that far better alternatives exist.

Of course, a diagnosis is not made on auscultation findings alone. A patient with shortness of breath, twenty-pound weight gain and lower extremity swelling who also has crackles is highly suggestive of pulmonary edema, even though auscultation alone has poor specificity. But why should we accept such poor diagnostic accuracy at all? Why, in the era of high definition TV, are we listening for signs of life-threatening illness on a staticky-radio-feed analog? Why are we using techniques developed at a time when the treatment of pneumonia was vile bark tonics, potent laxatives, and vein laceration to inflict "copious bleeding," of which Laennec thought was "productive of the most striking benefit"?[1]

Why must we continue to listen, infer, and guess what pathology is sitting within the chest when we can look inside and know for sure? It is time we pull our anachronistic diagnostic capabilities out of the 1800s and enter the *POCUS Era.*

CHAPTER 5: THE VIEW BETWEEN TWO RIBS

"In science, as well as in religion and politics, over-zealous and injudicious friends are often more injurious to the cause they advocate, than its most determined enemies; and in regard to auscultation, I am convinced that the most certain mode of preventing its general adoption, is to attempt to extend it beyond its just limits, or to raise its credit at the expense of other methods in more general use, which have not merely the sanction of the experience of ages, but the still stronger support of deep-rooted prejudice, in their favor."

DR. JOHN FORBES, 1827

Eight miles Northeast of *Necker Hospital* where Dr. Laennec rose to prominence more than 150 years prior sits *Delafontaine Hospital*, just blocks from Paris's George-Valbon State Park. In 1985 a young bright-eyed physician by the name of Daniel Alexandre Lichtenstein arrived for his first night shift in the intensive care unit there, scared and anxious of what could be.

As the night progressed, one of his patients was getting worse. A chest X-ray revealed a near white out of both lungs, a sign of impending respiratory doom. Yet was this pneumonia? Was it infectious fluid accumulating around the lungs and preventing them from expanding? The chest X-ray resolution was not sufficient to tell. When midnight struck and the radiologists left, Lichtenstein snuck into the radiology department, unplugged the ultrasound machine, and rolled it into the patient's room. He squirted ultrasound gel on the surface of the probe, gently placed it on the patient's flank, and the diagnosis revealed itself.

Centered on the ultrasound screen was a compressed lung gently bobbing up and down like a buoy in the ocean, completely surrounded by fluid. This **pleural effusion** was preventing the lung from expanding, and it needed to be drained urgently. It "was pleural tamponade. Inserting the needle was beneficial for the patient ... but please, consider that [using ultrasound at the bedside] was completely irregular and forbidden," he would later recount.[28]

At the time, "nobody did (or believed in) lung ultrasound," explained Lichtenstein, especially not at the patient's bedside. He had learned basic ultrasound techniques in 1984 at *Hospital Beaujon* from the famous French radiologist, Dr. Yves Menu.[29] It was an opportunity he pursued after witnessing a sonographic exam for the first time. "I fell in love with ultrasound ... I thought wow! What a scary but extraordinary tool. We can look inside, it's visual medicine."

A few years later he went to work at *Ambroise Pare Hospital* under the famed Dr. Francois Jardin. He chose this ICU "because it was the only ICU in the world which was equipped with ultrasound. We can say he created 'echocardiography in the ICU.'" It was exclusively used for cardiac ultrasound until Lichtenstein began experimenting with imaging of other portions of the body. "Before it was the current craze," he explained, "I introduced subclavian (or jugular) venous cannulation" with Jardin's ADR-4000, a large and clunky but functional ultrasound machine from the early 1980s.

It was here where Lichtenstein (Figure 4) would develop the field of bedside ultrasonography, hone his craft, and propel medicine into the *POCUS Era*. Just as Laennec validated his wheezes and crackles with autopsies, Lichtenstein corroborated various ultrasound findings with CT scans ordered by other clinicians.[3] Also like Laennec, he was intrinsically motivated to improve diagnostic accuracy to help his patients, staying up deep into the night scanning lung after lung while his co-workers slept. With each scan, he was trying to answer the question: "how to be useful to the patient?" And day by day, the field of point-of-care ultrasound was born.

As demonstrated on Lichtenstein's first ICU shift, a chest X-ray was not precise enough to detect the cause of shortness of breath in that patient. Ultrasound was. As Dr. Laennec two centuries earlier discovered a real-time audible window into the thorax, here now was a *visual window* into the entire body, offering a glimpse of the inner organs at work. This set Lichtenstein off on a journey to discover just how useful it may be.

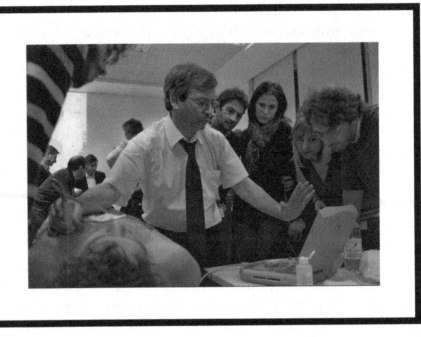

FIGURE 4   Dr. Daniel Lichtenstein, the trailblazer for modern day whole body point-of-care ultrasound. His studies proved how useful A-lines, B-lines, and lung sliding can be in diagnosing pulmonary disease. Pictured here teaching lung ultrasound.

Used with permission from Dr. Lichtenstein

Ultrasound basics

Sounds, by definition, are vibrations audible to the human ear,[30] made up of waves between 20 and 20,000 Hertz. This range varies by individual and deteriorates as we age.[31] Climbing higher into the sound spectrum reside *ultra* (Latin for 'beyond') sound waves, in the range of 2 to 18 Megahertz, inaudible to humans.[32]

In ultrasonography, these ultrasound waves are both emitted and received by an ultrasound probe. They are shot out at certain frequency ranges, travel through different tissues with varying degrees of ease, and reflect back to the probe at which point it integrates various wave characteristics to create a real-time image.

This sonar-inspired technology mimics what bats use to detect prey in the pitch black of night, submarines to traverse the deep sea, or even blind humans to navigate their surroundings with tongue clicking.[33] It has no ionizing radiation and has been used since as early as 1942, making it one of the safest forms of imaging that exists in the world today.

The ease or difficulty with which these sound waves traverse different parts of the body depends on the physical properties of the tissue. Ultrasound waves can pass well through the skin, adipose, or muscle, and therefore visualize these tissues and the structures deep to them quite well. They also travel well through fluid or pus filled structures like pleural effusions, full bladders, or pneumonias. However, this super-hero-like ability to look inside a human comes with its own kryptonite. One thing ultrasound cannot do well is penetrate through air. Due to the air's reflective properties, visualizing a structure behind an air-filled cavity is simply not possible, which is why as recently as 2008, *Harrison's Principles of Internal Medicine*, the seminal modern medical textbook, incorrectly reported that lungs are a major hindrance to ultrasound imaging.[34] The other tissue that ultrasound cannot see through is bone. Fortunately, nature has given us multiple windows into the thorax, between two ribs.

Pneumothorax & Lung Sliding

Situated in a vertical orientation between the ribs of the thorax are intercostal muscles that contract to expand the ribcage and assist with inspiration. The innermost layer of the thoracic wall is a slippery liner known as the *parietal pleura*. Much as two microscope slides stick together with a drop of water in between them, this parietal pleura connects to the lung's outermost surface, the *visceral pleura*, with a very fine layer of fluid to create a surface tension that allows them to slide past each other with each breath.[35] This sliding creates a bright, shimmering appearance on ultrasound, first seen in horses in 1986[36] and humans one year later.[37] As Dr. Lichtenstein first described it in a 1995 study:[38]

> "between two ribs, a hyperechogenic line, behind which only airy artifacts are present, is always visible ... this line is the interface between the soft tissues of the chest wall and the aerated lung. In a normal subject, one can identify at this lung-wall interface ... a kind of to-and-fro movement synchronized with respiration. This movement is striking because the surrounding structures are motionless, we may call it "pleural sliding" or perhaps a better term would be 'lung sliding.'"

When this parietal-visceral pleural seal is broken - usually due to air leaking between the lung and the internal thoracic wall - the lung collapses in that area like a partially deflated balloon and the lung sliding no longer occurs. Just like an air bubble in a snow globe, the less dense air will float to the top of the more dense liquid and sit in the part of the globe closest to the sky. This is precisely how a pneumothorax behaves. When the patient lies flat on their back, the air bubble sits anteriorly on top of the lungs just behind their ribs, the least dependent portion of the thorax.

Pneumothoraces are a significant problem especially in the intensive care unit,[39] and there are various ways to detect them. One is with a stethoscope, which involves listening for an absence of breath sounds since there is no lung inflation and deflation at that point. To some degree, this technique has stood the test of time; however, as already discussed it cannot distinguish a pneumothorax from a hemothorax or a pleural effusion. The stethoscope also cannot detect a small pneumothorax, and is further limited in the ICU, where lung auscultation is often rendered futile by the ventilator's rhythmic noises.

Another simple option is a chest X-ray. It is very useful for ruling in a pneumothorax with a specificity approaching 100%, however, its sensitivity to detect them can be as low as 28%.[40] While CT scan is the gold standard, this requires up to 500 chest-X-rays-worth of radiation[41] and the patient to be wheeled to a CT scanner, a luxury not afforded to many critically ill patients.

Ultimately, the problem with relying on a chest X-ray, versus a CT scan or ultrasound, is that the lungs are three-dimensional structures being assessed with a two-dimensional image. When the patient is on their back in a supine position, the air will travel to the anterior, least dependent portion of the lung, where chest X-ray has the lowest sensitivity for picking it up.[42] Especially in trauma patients or intubated patients, asking them to sit up to improve radiographic detection is not practical.

Prior to the 1990s, lung ultrasound was not considered an option to detect a pneumothorax because of its inability to visualize air-filled structures. Yet when Lichtenstein placed the ultrasound probe in the rib space corresponding to the pneumothorax seen on a CT scan in one of his studies, the lung sliding "was absent in all 41 analyzable pneumothoraces ... even in the case of a small anterior pneumothorax that was undetectable using chest radiography." If anterior lung sliding was present, then it ruled out pneumothorax 100% of the time, and if lung sliding was absent, it was 95% sensitive and 91% specific for pneumothorax.[38] These results were impressive, though not surprising to Lichtenstein since lung ultrasound is just visualizing the lung tissue itself. "Pneumothorax ultrasound will definitely be of the greatest value in critically ill patients," he exclaimed. "In this field, ultrasound should ideally be used routinely as a visual stethoscope."

Lung sliding, Lichtenstein argued, was a better test for pneumothorax. Yet other lung diseases that affect the pleura can also prevent lung sliding, such as focal pneumonias, surgical pneumothorax repairs like pleurodesis, acute respiratory distress syndrome, or pulmonary fibrosis. In these diseases, the parietal and visceral pleura are still approximating each other, however, they are not sliding as they should.

In addition to detecting a lack of lung sliding in a pneumothorax, Lichtenstein wondered if ultrasound could pinpoint the precise location where the detached portion of the lung re-attaches back to the chest wall. If this was the case, then the other diseases that prevent lung sliding could be ruled out as well.

While it is not seen in every pneumothorax (only 66% sensitive), this area of transition he dubbed the *lung point*,[43] was 100% specific to pneumothorax. It was "pathognomonic (that is, uniquely characteristic) of a pneumothorax," he later wrote, "and we can write this still today, 15 years after the publication of the lung point. We have never observed a lung point in the countless patients we visited who had no pneumothorax."[44]

There have been multiple large studies comparing the accuracy of lung ultrasound for pneumothorax detection against standard chest X-ray imaging, and almost all favor ultrasound (Table 1). In 2011, a meta-analysis out of a University Hospital in China including 20 studies found a pooled sensitivity and specificity of detecting pneumothorax with ultrasound at 89% and 99% respectively, compared to 50% and 100% respectively for chest X-rays.[45] A year later, a group of Canadian physicians did another meta-analysis examining eight studies and found nearly identical results.[46] Lastly, in 2013, researchers at Louisiana State University studied this as well, concluding that lung ultrasound was 78% sensitive and 98% specific, while chest X-rays were only 39% sensitive, confirming that lung ultrasound "remains much more sensitive than [chest X-ray] for identification of pneumothorax."[47]

These findings demonstrate that peering into each rib space and evaluating for lung sliding offers a glimpse of the lung's state of health. Below the shimmering pleura resides the lung tissue, filled with air and invisible to the ultrasound waves when functioning normally. What we also can see are sonographic artifacts that arise from the pleural line, which to the untrained eye appear to be useless noise.

	SENSITIVITY	SPECIFICITY
Stethoscope & Physical Exam	70%	99%*
Chest X-ray	28 - 75%	86 - 100%
POCUS	88%	99%

TABLE 1   **DIAGNOSING PNEUMOTHORAX**

Stethoscope & Physical Exam: Detecting absent breath sounds. *These numbers are misleading because they include hemothorax/pleural effusions. Also falsely inflated results since compared to chest x-ray. From Arts et al 2020.

Chest X-ray: Based on studies from literature review by Wilkerson et al 2009

POCUS: Adapted from meta-analysis by Ding et al 2011

A-lines & B-lines

When an object sits between two mirrors facing each other, an infinite number of reflections appear, with each image roughly equidistant from the previous. This is called the *infinity mirror effect*,[48] a phenomenon many first experience on the mirror-straddled pedestal in a department store fitting room. This reflective phenomenon is also seen when the ultrasound probe is placed between two ribs, causing either horizontal or vertical artifacts to emanate from the pleura. When the pleura is flat and dry, it emits *A-line* artifacts "reverberating at regular intervals, yielding parallel, roughly horizontal hyperechogenic lines," as Dr. Lichtenstein initially described them in 1997.[49] These *A-lines* are infinity-mirror-like reflections back and forth between the pleural line and the ultrasound probe (Figure 5). Intact lung sliding coupled with A-lines is the sonographic signature of normal lung tissue, what Lichtenstein called the *A-profile*. This duo can also be seen in certain diseases that do not distort the pleural line, such as COPD, asthma, or pulmonary embolism.

When the pleural line is jagged or wet, or both, it can also emit vertical projections called *B-lines* where "the beam seems to be "trapped" in a closed system, resulting in endless to-and-fro echoing," Lichtenstein noted, which manifests as "comet-tail artifacts" or spotlight projections shooting out of the pleura (Figure 5). And these B-lines, he observed, are absent under normal conditions.

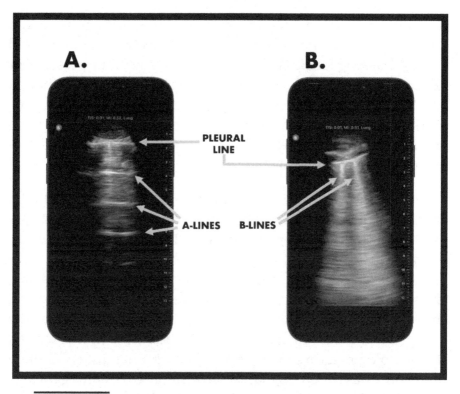

FIGURE 5 **A.** Example of A-lines, a sign of normal lung tissue. The first line is the lung sliding of the parietal and visceral pleura. The other lines are reflections.

B. Example of B-lines. When the pleura is wet or jagged, or both, from either pulmonary edema or infection, the interlobular septae swell and emit these spotlight projections. Two are pictured here. Lichtenstein coined the term *Lung Rockets* for three or more in a given rib space.

This comet-tail artifact was first described in 1982, arising from liver-embedded shotgun pellets[50] although its medical implications were not understood until the late 1990s when Lichtenstein began investigating whether this artifact carried any clinical significance in the lungs. Up until that time "no correlation [with the comet-tail artifacts] had been made with a pathologic feature. As a consequence, no practical use had been made from this artifact at the lung level."[51]

Lichtentein called these comet-tail artifacts arising from the lung pleura *B-lines*, which result from a "mingling of fluid and air" in the **interlobular septae**, the connective tissue in and around the lung lobes. This mingling happens in the presence of cardiogenic pulmonary edema or focal diseases like pneumonia. While singular B-lines can be seen in normal lungs, if three or more B-lines were present together in between a rib space, it was an abnormal finding he called a **lung rocket**, due to its resemblance to a spaceship at liftoff.

To test this hypothesis, Dr. Lichtenstein studied 282 patients admitted to the ICU over 18 months and what he found was impressive, definitive, and irrefutable. The lung rockets were almost exclusively present in areas of edema or infection.[51] He also observed that each B-line was roughly 7 millimeters apart, the same distance separating each interlobular septae seen on the corresponding CT scan. It was this study 15 years after the comet-tail artifact first appeared in the literature that described the pathologic nature of these B-lines in human lungs. Equally important was the confirmation that the absence of lung rockets was a sign of normal lung tissue. This provided further evidence that a lung ultrasound artifact showed tremendous diagnostic accuracy in an organ previously thought to be sonographically invisible. The potential for these findings was immense. Dr. Lichtenstein eventually devised seven criteria a vertical artifact must have to qualify as a B-line:[52]

1. It is always a comet-tail artifact or spotlight projection
2. It always arises from the pleural line
3. It always moves with lung sliding
4. It is almost always well defined, laser-like
5. It is almost always long and spreads to the edge of the screen
6. It almost always obliterates or obscures the A-lines
7. It is almost always hyperechoic, or bright

Lichtenstein applied this newly found knowledge to his patients with shortness of breath in another study, finding that "when compared to normal subjects, the lung surface appeared pathologic in pulmonary edema and normal in COPD." Lung rockets were seen in 100% of patients with pulmonary edema and absent in 92% of patients with COPD, a discovery that makes sense since COPD primarily affects the bronchioles and tissue of the lung and does not corrupt the pleural lining that ultrasound can visualize. "Screening for the comet-tail artifact arising from the pleural line," Lichtenstein concluded, "can help to distinguish between cardiogenic pulmonary edema and exacerbation of COPD ... It may thus contribute to quicker relief for dyspneic patients."[49]

Through his research challenging the status quo of the time, Lichtenstein showed that not only are these artifacts useful, but in fact map directly to various pulmonary diseases, much in the same way Laennec demonstrated with wheezes or rhonchi. As discussed in the coming chapters, Lichtenstein showed that just by using a standardized protocol to detect the absence or presence of lung sliding, A-lines, and B-lines, he could arrive at the correct diagnosis almost every time. Lung sliding combined with A-lines point to normal lung tissue and diseases that don't usually distort the pleura, such as pulmonary emboli, COPD, or asthma. In contrast, like a drug-sniffing dog alerting the authorities to cocaine-filled underwear, multiple lung rockets in the presence of normal lung sliding is highly suggestive of pulmonary edema.

CHAPTER 6: PULMONARY EDEMA & ULTRASOUND

"The treatment of congestion of the lungs is usually that of the condition with which it is associated. In the intense pulmonary engagement … free bleeding should be practised. From twenty to thirty ounces of blood should be taken from the arm, and if blood does not flow freely and the condition of the patient is desperate, aspiration of the right auricle (i.e. atrium) may be performed."

SIR WILLIAM OSLER, PRINCIPLES AND PRACTICE OF MEDICINE, 1892

The lung is a conically shaped, spongiform organ that takes up the majority of space inside the ribcage. Divided into 5 lobes, three on the right and two on the left, each lobe is divided into *lobules*, and each lobule is separated by connective tissue called *septae*, as discussed previously. Each lobule consists of millions of gas exchange units[53] called *alveoli* that are connected to the trachea by an ever-shrinking bronchial tree composed of about 1,500 miles worth of straw-like tubes that transport inhaled air from your mouth down to the deepest crevice of the lung and back out again on exhalation.[54]

Traveling alongside this bronchial tree is an arterial system, starting with the large pulmonary artery all the way down to the microscopic capillaries that surround the alveoli. It is at this microscopic level where gas exchange occurs. Like passengers at a busy train station, oxygen exits the alveoli and enters the capillaries while carbon dioxide exits the capillaries and enters the alveoli.

The alveoli and capillaries are separated by the *interstitial space*, which harbors small amounts of fluid dispersed throughout the tissue of healthy lungs. There is a homeostatic to-and-fro of fluid leakage from the capillaries into the interstitial space, however, it cannot enter the alveoli during normal conditions. The total amount of fluid outside the capillaries in this interstitial space is called the *Extravascular Lung Water* (from here on referred to as *lung water*), and it is strictly regulated to be about 500 milliliters by your lymphatic system, pouring any excess fluid back into the large veins for recirculation.[55]

Small fluctuations in this lung water can be controlled with this mechanism; however, beyond a certain threshold, this excess can quickly overwhelm the lymphatics. "In all forms of intense congestion," as famed physician and founding professor of Johns Hopkins Hospital Sir William Osler described it in 1892, "there is a transudation of serum from the engorged capillaries chiefly into the air cells, but also into the alveolar walls."[56] Like a clogged toilet that continues to fill, the excess fluid has nowhere else to go and overflows into the interstitial space, damaging the local alveoli in its wake.

It is this process of fluid build-up overwhelming insufficient lymphatic drainage and resulting alveolar injury that causes shortness of breath. It is also this plumbing failure and resulting irregular interlobular septae that project lung rockets and allow us to detect the edema. Since these capillaries are distributed all over the lung tissue, pulmonary edema due to cardiac causes is a diffuse pathologic process and distributes in both lungs evenly;

and since this type of edema is non-inflammatory in nature, it does not impair lung sliding. Therefore, if lung sliding is present along with lung rockets on both sides and in multiple rib spaces - what Lichtenstein called the *B-profile* - then it is almost certainly due to pulmonary edema.

Lung Rockets in Practice

In addition to qualitative detection, we know that lungs projecting lung rockets in two or more rib spaces have more excess lung water than average. Likewise, lungs without evidence of lung rockets are 90% sensitive and specific for normal amounts of lung water.[57] We also know that the number of B-lines do increase with worsening shortness of breath[58] and disappear with appropriate treatment, either with diuretics[59] or hemodialysis.[60,61]

When Canadian physicians used Lichtenstein's findings to evaluate patients presenting to the emergency department with shortness of breath, lung ultrasound was 93% sensitive for detecting pulmonary edema cases while chest X-rays were only 63% sensitive.[62] These results were similar to a Turin, Italy emergency department study, where the sensitivity and specificity of lung rockets was 93% and 84% respectively.[63]

A few years later in Slovenia, 218 patients presenting to the emergency department with shortness of breath were evaluated with lung ultrasound as well. In an exam that "was always under 1 minute," patients with lung rockets in two or more rib spaces were considered positive for pulmonary edema. They also recorded whether the patient had orthopnea (shortness of breath when lying flat), whether they heard rales when listening with a stethoscope, and checked an NT-proBNP blood test, which is elevated in patients with heart failure.

They calculated the odds of having pulmonary edema if one of the above factors was positive. For rales, the odds ratio was 5.1, meaning the odds of having pulmonary edema if rales are present is 5.1 times that of someone without rales present. For orthopnea, it was 6.9. For elevated NT-proBNP it was 14.3, while for lung rockets in two or more rib spaces, the odds of having pulmonary edema was a whopping *53.7 times* those without lung rockets, concluding that "ultrasound examination was the single best method for confirming the diagnosis of acute [heart failure] in the prehospital setting."[64]

These results were consistent with a large Italian study in 2015, where they found that "a lung ultrasound-implemented approach had a higher diagnostic accuracy than other commonly used diagnostic tools," with sensitivity and specificity of 97%, compared to 69% and 82% respectively with chest X-ray.[65] Such impressive diagnostic accuracy is consistent with the findings of three meta-analyses in 2014, 2018, and 2019,[66–68] solidifying Dr. Lichtenstein's work as a crucial foundation for the *POCUS Era*, and providing clinicians with an enormously powerful tool to differentiate causes of shortness of breath at the bedside (Table 2).

	SENSITIVITY	SPECIFICITY
Stethoscope & Physical Exam	64%	67%
Chest X-ray	63%	93%
POCUS	97%	98%

TABLE 2 **DIAGNOSING PULMONARY EDEMA**

Stethoscope & Physical Exam: Detecting crackles. Adapted from Arts et al 2020.

Chest X-ray: Study of emergency department patients. Nakao et al 2021

POCUS: Detecting lung rockets in two or more rib spaces. From meta-analysis by Wang et al 2018

CHAPTER 7: PNEUMONIA & ULTRASOUND

"The Russian who rolls himself in the snow after coming out of the hot bath, or the baker who goes from his heated oven, almost naked, into an atmosphere of a temperature below zero, is not liable to attacks of this disease: while the porters, whose occupation leads them to stand for a length of time at the corners of the streets, are frequently affected by it. In general, pneumonia is a disease of winter and cold climates: it is rare in the equatorial regions. The poison of serpents, particularly that of the rattle-snake, frequently induces this disease, and the same result follows the injection of various medicamentous substances into the veins."

DR. LAENNEC DESCRIBING PNEUMONIA, 1819

Just deep to the lung sliding visualized in each rib space lies the lung tissue itself. When sections of the lung become inflamed or infected and fill with fluid or pus it can form a *lung consolidation,* and this portion of the lung previously veiled with air, becomes visible to ultrasound. In fact, to some degree, the ultrasound can visualize lung tissue in direct proportion to the level of disease that exists in that area, assuming it approximates the pleura, which is the case more than 98% of the time.[69] This process of consolidation of a portion of the lung is called *hepatization,* due to its resemblance to liver, or hepatic, tissue. The lung "has entirely lost its crepitous feel under the finger, and has acquired a consistence and weight altogether resembling those of liver,"[1] as Laennec described it from one of his autopsies.

Whether in an outpatient clinic, urgent care, or hospital setting, a chest X-ray is routinely ordered to evaluate a patient presenting with shortness of breath or cough. If this chest X-ray does not detect a lung consolidation (also known as an *opacity*), then it is often assumed that the patient does not have pneumonia; however, this is not necessarily the case.

In a study looking at 97 patients presenting to the hospital with respiratory symptoms, chest X-rays missed 27% of cases of pneumonia that were found on gold-standard CT scans,[70] while another study of 188 febrile, immunosuppressed patients found that 60% of them had CT findings of pneumonia with a normal corresponding chest X-ray.[71] Researchers at Vanderbilt University studied over 3,400 patients and found that chest X-rays missed over half of pneumonias seen on CT scans, while only one-quarter of the patients with chest X-rays interpreted by the radiologist as having pneumonia actually did. The researchers concluded that chest X-rays "cannot independently rule-in or rule-out pneumonia,"[72] and that given the millions of annual emergency department visits for respiratory symptoms, "an 'opacity equals antibiotics' reflexive management strategy is likely to lead to frequent overuse of antibiotics and unnecessary pressure for the development of antibiotic resistance."

These are the dangers of low-performance screening tests. Like Gunther's rusty lobster cage accidentally catching tuna fish, a chest X-ray may falsely detect pneumonia and inappropriately trigger antibiotics. Likewise, just as Gunther's rudimentary lobster trap didn't catch 30% of the lobsters, pneumonia not detected by chest X-ray would go untreated. This is not to say that chest X-rays do not serve a large purpose. Suspicious findings can prompt a CT scan or other higher resolution imaging studies. However, the limitations of an X-ray's two-dimensional nature must be understood to appropriately interpret the results.

Even if a clinician wanted to instead order a lung ultrasound for a patient, in most hospitals it is still not possible. Strangely, ultrasound studies can be ordered for veins, arteries, livers, kidneys, spleens, bladders, or hearts, but not for the lungs. Likely based on the outdated thinking that lung ultrasound is not feasible, a chest X-ray is still the standard first choice of lung imaging despite its poor sensitivity.

A chest X-ray of the lungs is analogous to a photograph of a large pine tree. It is a static two-dimensional snapshot in time that portrays a triangular-shaped tree with spiky-green-pine-covered branches emerging from the trunk. The trunk of the tree may be visualized through the more sparse portions while hidden through the dense ones. But it would not portray a light breeze displacing the branches every few seconds, or an animal nesting in the back.

In comparison, lung ultrasound is a series of semi-immediate dynamic snippets of lung tissue separated by ribs. It is more like a drone-mounted video camera, traveling around the pine tree in horizontal circles as it makes its way down the trunk. Unlike the photograph, this drone can appreciate the real-time subtle movement of the tree branches, as well as any animals that may be dwelling in the back. Like a pointillist painting of your respiratory organ, these snippets of ultrasound can then be mentally pieced together to form a three-dimensional image of the lung.

Focal Lung Rockets, Shred Sign & PLAPS

Lichtenstein convincingly demonstrated that cardiogenic pulmonary edema causes the interlobular septae to swell and emit lung rockets across multiple rib spaces. He characterized this type of non-infectious, non-inflammatory fluid present with the B-profile as "a lubricant which does not impair lung sliding."[44] Yet when edema from inflammation or infection fills the alveoli and the interlobular septae swell, lung rockets appear as well; however, they are often focused in discrete regions of the lung and lung sliding commonly becomes impaired (what he called the *B-prime profile*). This *exudative* fluid as it is called, "is a biologic glue. We assume that each exudative B-line acts as a *nail*. Since B-lines are numerous, these multiple nails should appear sufficient for sticking the lung to the wall." Such conditions arise in diseases like acute respiratory distress syndrome, pulmonary fibrosis or COVID-19 pneumonia, where lung rockets are present but lung sliding is often impaired. This flavor of absent lung sliding differs from that in pneumothorax by the presence of B-lines. Therefore, if B-lines are present, a pneumothorax can be ruled out.

In addition to focal lung rockets, if a consolidation is present it can often be visualized deep to the pleural line in the lung tissue itself. By nature of the erratic accumulation of fluid, pus, or irregular cells that occurs during the normal course of an infection or a cancer, consolidations that occupy a portion of the lung will have irregular, shredded borders with underlying normal lung deep to it. This is called the *shred sign*, and it can be used to identify a consolidation when it is seen (Figure 6).[52] The vast majority of these consolidations reside towards the base of the lung on the posterior-lateral side, a point Lichtentein dubbed the the *PLAPS point*, an acronym for the *posterolateral alveolar and/ or pleural syndrome point* mouthful.

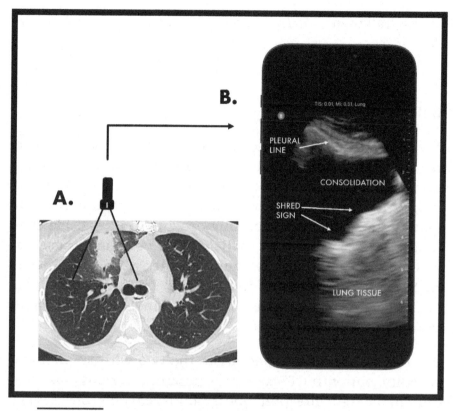

FIGURE 6   **A.** CT scan showing right lung consolidation

B. Corresponding ultrasound image. From top to bottom is skin & soft tissue, then the pleural line. Below the pleural line is a hypoechoic (dark) consolidation. The posterior wall of the consolidation has an irregular, jagged border, called the **shred sign**

But a lung ultrasound exam takes experience, time, and effort. Though usually completed in under five minutes, positioning the patient, adjusting the bed, applying the gel, acquiring the images, and interpreting them is more labor-intensive than clicking the *Order Chest X-ray* button in the electronic medical record. Within minutes to hours of placing such an order, a radiology technician appears at the bedside and takes an X-ray that is digitally transported into the radiologist's bloated to-be-read image queue. In due time the radiologist interprets the image and offers a final read, often including the following cringe-inducing statement: *"Atelectasis versus pneumonia, clinically correlate."*

Atelectasis Versus Pneumonia

The convenience and expedience of a chest X-ray come with the drawback of low resolution and its resulting ambiguous interpretations. This is especially true in the case of differentiating *atelectasis*, or partial lung collapse, from pneumonia. "The accurate causal diagnosis of lung opacities on a bedside chest radiograph ... is a frequent challenge. Two common causes are pneumonia and atelectasis," wrote Lichtenstein. Like a deflating balloon, the atelectasis is caused by "bronchial block to air entry," resulting in a contraction of the lung tissue, more aptly named *resorptive atelectasis*.

It is often difficult to differentiate the two with any imaging modality, but with CT scans or ultrasound, various clues may point in the right direction. One is Hounsfield units on CT scans, which are a measure of the relative brightness of each structure. Atelectasis tends to have higher Hounsfield units, and a value under 92 can accurately predict pneumonia with 97% sensitivity and 85% specificity.[73]

Meanwhile ultrasound's ability to distinguish pneumonia from atelectasis "comes first from its ability to document alveolar consolidation," Lichtenstein explained, which reaches the visceral pleura in over 98% of consolidations "creating the mandatory acoustic window for their ultrasound demonstration." Enclosed in these consolidations may be linear, branching portions of the bronchial tree now visible due to the surrounding edema called *air bronchograms*. Air bubbles inside these bronchioles can sometimes be seen moving up and down with each breath, indicating "preserved patency of the airways because the gas bubbles are pushed toward the end of the bronchi." These moving air bubbles are called *dynamic air bronchograms,* and they are seen in pneumonia, while *static air bronchograms*, that don't move at all, can be seen in both pneumonia and resorptive atelectasis.[74]

Lichtenstein felt these sonographic findings make ultrasound "useful every time the origin of a consolidation is unclear ... as an ultrasound shows not only the consolidation, as would radiograph or CT scan, but also a dynamic sign of clinical relevance ... it indicates that this consolidation is probably a pneumonia." Being able to watch the lung contract and expand as the patient breathes in and out, he continued, is also "one major advantage of ultrasonography compared to traditional imaging approaches such as radiography or CT scan, which cannot demonstrate lung expansion in real time."

Lichtenstein studied 52 patients with proven pneumonia compared to 16 with proven resorptive atelectasis. Dynamic air bronchograms had a 94% specificity and a 97% positive predictive value for diagnosing pneumonia and distinguishing it from resorptive atelectasis. "Lung ultrasonography's utility has been confirmed by a growing number of studies," he asserted as his research was gaining momentum, "and is simple to perform, provided one thinks differently."

Ruling In & Out Pneumonia

Ultrasound protocols to evaluate for pneumonia vary but generally involve looking at multiple rib spaces in both lungs, usually two anterior, one or two lateral, and the PLAPS point looking for impaired lung sliding, focal lung rockets, or lung consolidations. A 2020 study in a Minneapolis, Minnesota ICU found that when compared with gold standard CT scans, using a similar protocol detected up to 92.5% of consolidations as compared to only 65.7% with chest X-ray.[75] Another study of Chinese patients with community-acquired pneumonia showed that lung ultrasound and chest X-rays had sensitivities of 94% and 77% respectively, with similar specificities.[76] This superiority of lung ultrasound for detecting pneumonia has been confirmed in Dutch kids under 16 years old,[77] in Chinese neonates,[78] in Greek ICU patients,[79] in adults with COVID-19 pneumonia,[80] and even in patients presenting to a remote emergency department in Nepal.[81] With sensitivities and specificities in the 90% range,[82] this pocket-sized device can rule in or rule out pneumonia with near certainty. Validated by multiple meta-analyses,[82,83] this research begs the question why lung ultrasound, with its zero ionizing radiation icing-on-the-cake, is not the first line pulmonary imaging option for all patients (Table 3).

	SENSITIVITY	SPECIFICITY
Stethoscope & Physical Exam	33%	87%
Chest X-ray	43%	93%
POCUS	85-95%	93-98%

TABLE 3 **DIAGNOSING PNEUMONIA**

Stethoscope & Physical Exam: Adapted from Arts et al 2020. Findings compared to chest X-ray which artificially inflates results.

Chest X-ray: Adapted from Self et al 2013.

POCUS: From two meta-analyses: Alzahrani et al 2017 and Balk et al 2017

Nowhere is such diagnostic accuracy needed more than in the outpatient setting. In Europe for example, as much as 90% of antibiotics are prescribed by general practitioners, the majority of which are for suspected respiratory tract infections.[84] In a clinic environment with no access to immediate imaging and no good screening tests, the decision to prescribe antibiotics is largely subjective, ultimately leading to excess antibiotic use and resistance.

There are many contributors to the antibiotic overprescription problem, including patient expectations or medical-legal repercussions; however, it is fundamentally a function of poor screening tests. If there was a nasal swab or blood test that could say with over 90% sensitivity and specificity that the patient did or did not have pneumonia, then this would not be such a problem. While we don't have such a laboratory test, we do have lung ultrasound with similarly impressive diagnostic capabilities, yet it is rarely or ever evoked as a method for narrowing our antibiotic use for respiratory infections. One can only speculate how many fewer antibiotics we would use, how much antibiotic resistance we could spare, or how much radiation exposure could be averted if we follow the protocols developed by Dr. Lichtenstein and used our ultrasound probe in place of our stethoscope when examining a patient with respiratory symptoms.

CHAPTER 8: PLEURAL
EFFUSIONS & ULTRASOUND

"The fluctuation of the fluid in the right cavity of the chest was very perceptible, on succussion, after death ... when punctured an elastic fluid escaped from it with a hissing noise...There was found in the vacity of the pleura a considerable quantity of sero-purulent liquid, of a greenish-yellow colour, very frothy on the surface, and semi-transparent, not withstanding the great portion of puriform fragments that floated in it."

DR. LAENNEC DESCRIBING A CASE OF LETHAL RIGHT EM-
PYEMA, 1819

Whether in pulmonary edema or pneumonia, fluid can leak out of the lung and accumulate in the thorax resulting in a pleural effusion. In contrast to the air in a pneumothorax, this fluid collects in the lowest, *most dependent* portion of the thorax. Therefore, in a patient sitting upright, the fluid will collect around the base of the lungs, above the diaphragm. This fluid accumulation can prevent the lung from expanding, termed **compressive atelectasis**, and no breath sounds would be heard close to the base of the lung. However, when trying to detect this fluid on a physical exam, classically taught findings like Auenbrugger's dullness to percussion or Laennec's decreased breath sounds have very limited effectiveness.[85] Percussion only penetrates to a maximum depth of 6cm, limiting its use in overweight or obese patients, and cannot reliably detect an effusion less than 300 milliliters.[86]

The ultimate question though is *what to do with the information that there may be a pleural effusion*. How much fluid is in there? Is it one big pocket of free fluid, or separated into multiple compartments? Does it need to be drained? Is there pneumonia as well? Is it a **transudative** effusion, caused by congestive heart failure, or more likely to be **exudative**, resulting from cancer or infection?

As with any other pulmonary disease, the traditional first step is a chest X-ray. As demonstrated in Lichtenstein's first intensive care unit night shift however, this two-dimensional image has poor sensitivity and specificity for pleural effusions, especially if there are multiple pathologies present at once. Yet even with just a clear-cut pleural effusion, at least 200 milliliters of fluid needs to accumulate before a chest X-ray can even detect it, with sensitivities ranging from 33-92%.[86] Meanwhile, ultrasound can detect effusions as small as three milliliters[87] and is 100% sensitive for effusions over 100 milliliters.[88] When the patient is sitting upright, the effusion is at its largest yet chest X-ray can mistake them for lung consolidations,[89] or completely miss as many as 10% of effusions large enough to be drained.[90] Lichtenstein believed that with ultrasound guidance, even effusions too small to be visualized on chest X-ray could be successfully drained to expedite a patient's recovery. He demonstrated this in a study of 44 patients with thoracentesis-proven pleural effusions, finding that chest X-rays missed 17 of them and labeled another 6 as "possible," while lung ultrasound detected all 44.[91]

If the patients are lying flat on their back, X-rays are even worse.[86] Like a half-filled water bottle when placed on its side, the fluid will spread from the diaphragm area towards the head and collect along the posterior ribs. In this position, one study found chest X-rays falsely detected an effusion in 20% of patients who did not have one, missed 30% of effusions less than 300 milliliters, and missed one case of a pleural effusion over 1,200 milliliters.[92]

As far back as 1976 in Warsaw, Poland, researchers already thought ultrasound imaging was better than chest X-ray for detecting pleural effusions. "Radiologic examination has, so far, been the commonly used method of detecting pleural effusions," they wrote in a study of 116 patients with pleural effusions, "however, a routine posteroanterior chest roentgenogram [that is, chest X-ray] may not reveal the fluid in cases of small pleural effusion."[87] Ultrasound had better sensitivity, fewer false negatives, and didn't miss any effusions over 50 milliliters. "For the first time a comparison of the ultrasonic and radiologic methods has been made," they wrote in their conclusion, "and the superiority of the ultrasonic over the radiologic has been demonstrated." Lichtenstein's work corroborated this high accuracy of lung ultrasound, detecting pleural effusions with 92% sensitivity and 93% specificity in a study of ICU patients, compared to 39% and 85% respectively with a chest X-ray.[24] Such results have been duplicated in multiple modern-day studies,[93-95] confirming that lung ultrasound can rule in or rule out pleural effusions with near certainty (Table 4).

	300 MILLILITERS OR MORE		LESS THAN 300 MILLILITERS	
	SENSITIVITY	SPECIFICITY	SENSITIVITY	SPECIFICITY
Stethoscope & Physical Exam	46%	67%	CANNOT DETECT	CANNOT DETECT
One View Chest X-ray	33-82%	76-89%	CANNOT DETECT	CANNOT DETECT
POCUS	92-100%	88-100%	92-100%	88-100%

TABLE 4   DIAGNOSING PLEURAL EFFUSION

Stethoscope & Physical Exam: Dullness to percussion was best exam technique. Compared to a chest x-ray which cannot detect effusions under 300 milliliters which inflate results. Percussion limited in obese patients, only penetrates 6 cm. Adapted from Soni et al 2015.

Chest X-ray: Anterior to posterior chest X-rays when compared to thoracentesis or CT scan. Adapted from Soni et al 2015.

POCUS: Can detect effusion as small as 3 milliliters (Gryminski et al) through reliably over 20 milliliters. Over 100 milliliters it its about 100% sensitive and specific. Adapted from Soni et al 2015.

Spine sign, Jellyfish sign, Curtain sign

As compared to dullness to percussion or decreased breath sounds, in the *POCUS Era* there are three commonly used sonographic signs to diagnose a pleural effusion. When an ultrasound probe is placed on the side of a patient with a pleural effusion, if the fluid is pitch-black or **anechoic**, it can appear indistinguishable from air. Yet contrary to air, ultrasound waves travel very effectively through this fluid and brighten any structure sitting deep to it, which is why women are asked to fill their bladder before undergoing their routine pregnancy sonogram. With pleural effusions, these ultrasound waves travel to the patient's back and illuminate the thoracic spine. This is called the *spine sign*, and it is a clever way to differentiate effusions from a large pneumothorax. Bobbing up and down in this fluid can be a portion of the compressed lung that can look like a jellyfish swimming in the ocean hence termed the *jellyfish sign* (Figure 7).

Lastly is the *curtain sign*, which describes the lung expanding as it fills with air and washes over the ultrasound screen from the head towards the feet like a curtain. In a patient with a normal lung compressed with fluid, this can be seen with each inspiration.[96] Using these basic ultrasound techniques, pleural effusions can be detected with sensitivity and specificity approaching 100%, far better than can be achieved with lung auscultation or chest X-ray.

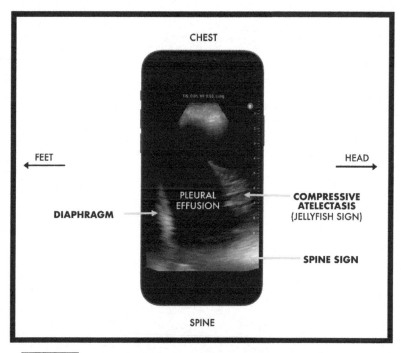

FIGURE 7   View of pleural effusion from lateral chest with patient supine. Feet are to the left, head is to the right. The diaphragm should be visualized when orienting the probe. If it is a true pleural effusion, there should be a *spine sign* present, since ultrasound waves can traverse the fluid and highlight any posterior structures. Floating in the fluid is a compressed lung that can look like a jellyfish.

CHAPTER 9: ELIMINATING CHEST X-RAYS

"We believe this 'ultrasound stethoscope' is very useful for the differential diagnosis ... it allows quick screening of ill patients with doubtful physical symptoms and signs since visualization of intra-abdominal organs or processes is readily available. The instrument can therefore be considered as an "extended palpation" ... Immediate and on-the-spot assessment of patients is now possible with this miniaturized, self-contained and battery powered ultrasound device ... It is expected that this miniaturized and automated instrument will have an important impact on the diagnostic use of ultrasound and the further development of ultrasonic equipment."

DR. JOS ROELANDT, ERASMUS UNIVERSITY, 1978

The average American is exposed to about three millisieverts (mSv) of radiation per year, either from radioactive radon gas in our homes, or from the cosmic radiation beaming down from the atmosphere. This exposure increases as the altitude rises, so a person living in Colorado at 3,300 feet has an annual radiation exposure that is slightly higher than someone living in Washington D.C., at only 410 feet above sea level. Interestingly though, the cancer risk at high altitude is not higher, and may even be lower.[97]

In comparison, a chest X-ray exposes a patient to 0.1 mSv and a mammogram to 0.4 mSv of ionizing radiation, which is about how much an average person would be exposed to naturally over the course of 10 days or 40 days respectively.[98] CT scans emit more ionizing radiation, ranging anywhere from 2 to 20 mSv depending on the type and location of the body scanned. This is roughly 20 to 200 times more than a chest X-ray, though still well below the United States occupational recommended annual radiation limit of 50 mSv.[99] However, when multiple CT scans are performed on a given patient, this limit can be breached and cancer risk can increase. For example, in a study of over 31,000 patients over 22 years, one-third underwent five or more lifetime CT scans and 5% underwent between 22 and 132 scans, resulting in up to a 12% excess lifetime risk of developing cancer above the baseline cancer incidence of 42%. However, the increased risk of the entire patient population included in the study was only 0.7%.[100]

CT scans are a miracle of medical science and have saved millions of lives, especially in urgent situations when the speed and accuracy of such imaging are essential. Yet a major disadvantage is the excess ionizing radiation exposure, a risk that is not well appreciated in the medical community. In a survey of emergency medicine physicians and radiologists, about 75% of the entire group significantly underestimated the radiation dose from a CT scan, and 53% of the radiologists and 91% of the emergency-room physicians did not believe that CT scans increased the lifetime risk of cancer.[101] This lack of appreciation may in part explain why CT scans are ordered so cavalierly.

Preventing unnecessary CT scans or X-rays is especially important in children since cancer risks related to radiation exposure decrease as people age. One study estimated that the risk of death from cancer from a single abdominal CT scan in a one-year-old is 1 in 550, and roughly 1 in 1500 for a head CT, which are "an order of magnitude higher than risks for adults."[102] This is due to the fact that children have more dividing cells and more years of life during which a potential cancer can develop.[103] Because of these facts, the United States annual federal dose limit for radiation exposure for those under 18 years old is only 5 mSv, 1/10th of that for an adult.[99] This is an upper limit that is unfortunately quite achievable with only one or two CT scans in a year.

According to the National Cancer Institute, the number of CT scans in children has increased 8-fold since 1980 resulting in 5 to 9 million performed annually.[104] With advancing CT scanners and increased awareness to the children's risk, the ionizing radiation exposure per scan is less and less, yet it is still between 2 and 9 mSv per scan according to one study of 200,000 kids.[105] While these risks are real, it is important to stress that the absolute cancer risks are still extremely small, and in many cases a CT scan provides essential information that cannot be practically obtained otherwise. Yet especially in children, any imaging modality that does not expose patients to ionizing radiation should first be considered.

With the strength of the data supporting lung ultrasound thus far, it is curious why it has not become first-line lung imaging and made chest X-rays less relevant. While most clinicians have not yet adapted to the *POCUS Era*, a hospital in China offers a glimpse into what an ultrasound-focused, radiation-free medical utopia might look like.

Zero Millisievert ICU

With concerns of excess radiation exposure, between 2017 and 2020, the Neonatal Intensive Care Unit at the Chaoyang District Maternal and Child Healthcare Hospital in Beijing, China abolished the use of chest X-rays completely, relying exclusively on lung ultrasound.

All infants underwent a complete lung ultrasound on admission to the ICU, if they improved or deteriorated, and upon discharge. Over the three-year-period they studied over 3,700 infants, about half of whom had a lung disease that prompted an ICU admission. Of those with lung disease, 269 had a chest X-ray at another hospital right before coming to their ICU, the results of which were often discordant to their ultrasound findings.

In one case, a chest X-ray mistakenly diagnosed a right upper lobe pneumonia in a newborn which ultrasound revealed was actually an enlarged thymus gland. In a baby admitted two hours after birth with a rapid breathing rate, a chest X-ray diagnosed her with a condition called *respiratory distress syndrome*. However, her lung ultrasound showed it was actually a small pneumothorax, and her condition improved once the air was removed. In another case, a patient was admitted 12 days after birth with fever and cough. The chest X-ray revealed normal lungs while the lung ultrasound clearly showed pneumonia, and the patient improved with antibiotics.

Overall the chest X-ray was consistent with the lung ultrasound 65% of the time, misdiagnosed 72 patients, and completely missed the diagnosis in 21 of them. An enlarged thymus was misdiagnosed as atelectasis in 12 patients, while the other misses included eleven cases of pneumonia, six cases of pneumothorax, and four pleural effusions.

During these three years in Beijing, the physicians proudly proclaimed that "none of the newborn infants hospitalized in the NICU of our hospital have undergone chest X-ray examination. All patients were diagnosed or had lung disease excluded by lung ultrasound examination. As a result, all hospitalized patients completely avoided radiation damage." This is in stark contrast to a typical neonatal ICU, where children can receive up to 30 chest X-rays in a given stay.[106] The authors felt their experience opens the door to "the 'new era of green diagnostics' for neonatal diseases," and proves that it is possible for an entire medical unit to completely replace chest X-rays with lung ultrasound.[78]

Lichtenstein's Lasting Impact

Part I of this book clearly demonstrates the power POCUS has over stethoscopes and chest X-rays for diagnosing diseases of the lung, a herculean tribute to Dr. Lichtenstein's innovative research. In what seems like the ultimate test of his life's work, 260 ICU patients with shortness of breath were evaluated by Lichtenstein and his colleagues in accordance with the lung ultrasound protocol he developed (Figure 8). Following this **BLUE Protocol**, and without knowing anything about the patients, he was able to arrive at the correct diagnosis in 90% of cases,[107] truly a remarkable feat from a previously overlooked method of lung imaging.

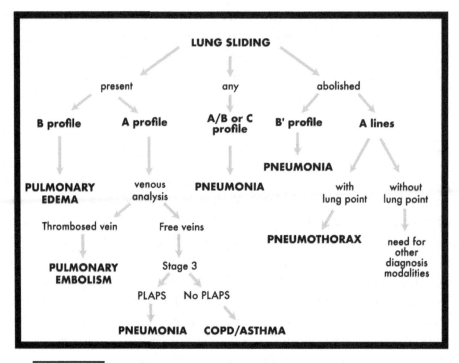

FIGURE 8   The Bedside Lung Ultrasound in Emergency (BLUE) Protocol. The culmination of Lichtenstein's research in lung ultrasound, which arrived at the correct diagnosis 90.5% of the time in 301 patients over 4 years.

Adapted from Lichtenstein et al 2008
Via https://bit.ly/3mnXgNa

When he started lung ultrasound, cardiac ultrasound was done by cardiologists and gynecologic ultrasound went to the OB-GYNs, while "the rest of the body was quietly given to the radiologists. The advent of lung ultrasound, a field ignored (and perhaps rejected) by experts from the beginning, has changed the landscape,"[108] he wrote. From pneumothorax to pneumonia, pleural effusions to edema, Lichtenstein proved that lung sliding, A-lines, and B-lines are today what Lannec's wheezes, rhonchi, and rales were two centuries ago. While he is most well known for his work with lung ultrasound, through his perseverance and dedication Lichtenstein pioneered the concept of examining the whole body with ultrasound at the bedside, what we refer to as POCUS today.

There are a number of striking similarities between Laennec and Lichtenstein. Both trained in Paris, spent time at Necker hospital, were passionate advocates for improving diagnostic accuracy, and developed a novel field of bedside diagnostics that launched medicine into a new era. Just as Laennec faced pushback with the advent of his stethoscope, Lichtenstein was met with ample criticism when introducing his new techniques to the medical field. It came from reviewers repeatedly rejecting his manuscripts, or from readers of his published articles. The criticism was everything from "why it cannot work, why it is impossible," to others saying if it were true, then why was it not known already? One colleague told him he would pay attention "once the radiologists would pay attention."

But the criticisms were not as bad as being ignored by prominent doctors in the field, he explained, who did not acknowledge his work, not caring to come up with an argument against lung ultrasound. "Someone told me," he said tongue-in-cheek in an interview, that "the most difficult part of research is the first 50 years. After that, everything gets simpler." Lichtenstein understands much of the pushback around using lung ultrasound in place of a stethoscope. "The stethoscope is the symbol of medicine. Scientifically speaking, ultrasound works better, no doubt. But emotionally, it is less simple. And we all have made medical decisions based on emotional stimulations."[29]

Lichtenstein would eventually have the last laugh, as his work has now been confirmed in multiple studies around the world and recommended by international guidelines.[109] This global corroboration has solidified him as the modern-day Laennec, the father of lung ultrasound, and probably the most influential early trailblazer dragging the field of bedside diagnostic medicine into the *POCUS era*.

PART II

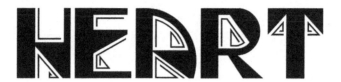

HEART

"A doctor, eh?" cried he, much excited. "Have you your stethoscope? Might I ask you - would you have the kindness? I have grave doubts as to my mitral valve, if you would be so very good. The aortic I may rely upon, but I should value your opinion upon the mitral."

I listened to his heart as requested, but was unable to find anything amiss, save indeed that he was in an ecstasy of fear, for he shivered from head to foot. "It appears to be normal," I said. "You have no cause for uneasiness."

"You will excuse my anxiety, Miss Morstan," he remarked airily. "I am a great sufferer, and I have long had suspicions as to that valve. I am delighted to hear that they are unwarranted."

SHERLOCK HOLMES, 1890

The Sign of the Four, A. Conan Doyle

INTRODUCTION

I n some ways, the heart was engineered for auscultation. While pneumonia alters the lung's outward appearance, just as a stab wound disfigures the skin, the afflictions affecting the heart modify the sound it emits rather than the look it maintains. From Laennec's walnut cylinder to Littman's dual earpiece stethoscope, two centuries of incremental improvements solidified into the art and science of cardiac auscultation, diagnosing millions of pathologies in the process. Yet with the advent of pocket-sized ultrasound devices, bright lights of scrutiny have converged upon auscultation's abilities and limitations as they compare to POCUS in various head-to-head studies.

Such a duel was staged at Cedar Sinai Medical Center in 2005, examining how brand new medical students with no clinical experience, outfitted with a handheld ultrasound and minimal training, would stack up against seasoned cardiologists with a stethoscope. The objective was simple: *who could diagnose common diseases of the heart more accurately?* Equipped with 18 hours of training, and without knowing anything about the patients, the medical students were asked to ultrasound each subject's heart. The cardiologists - who were also blinded to the known diagnoses - examined the same patients with their physical exam and stethoscope, and the results were another blow to the *Before POCUS Era*.

The students correctly identified 75% of pathologies while the cardiologists only found half. The students only missed 4% of "severe" cases while the cardiologists missed 32%. For all diseases of the heart valves, the first-year medical students picked up about 90% of them compared to 50% by the cardiologists, an especially large discrepancy in the case of *diastolic murmurs* where students detected 76% while cardiologists heard only 16% of them.[110]

The most important finding, the authors explained, is that the "diagnostic accuracy of first-year medical students using bedside cardiac ultrasound examinations was significantly superior to that of board-certified cardiologists performing cardiac physical examinations for the detection and evaluation of selected valvular and nonvalvular cardiac abnormalities." These differences, they insisted, "do not imply deficiency on the part of cardiologists," as multiple other studies on heart auscultation have found similarly poor diagnostic abilities, "but rather the great inherent difficulty involved in evaluating the function of many organs by use of palpation, percussion, and auscultation."

There are many valid arguments for the continued use of a stethoscope for cardiac auscultation. Yet if medical students with minimal experience and an ultrasound can outperform expert cardiologists with a stethoscope, is it time to admit that POCUS should become the protagonist while our trusty analog listening device assumes the supporting role?

CHAPTER 10: ECHOS
FROM WITHIN

"Blood is prepared in the liver, and is thence transferred to the heart to receive its proper form and last perfection a statement which does not appear devoid of reason; for no great, and perfect work is ever accomplished at a single effort, or receives its final polish from one instrument. But if this be actually so, then show us another vessel which draws the absolutely perfect blood from the heart, and distributes it as the arteries do the spirits over the whole body."

GALEN OF PERGAMON, ANCIENT GREEK PHYSICIAN CIRCA
129-217

Sitting just left of center in the thorax resides the heart, an impressive fist-sized organ that pumps blood to every inch of the body, including to itself, about three billion times in a lifespan. This number of heartbeats is remarkably preserved between species, ranging from the Galapagos tortoise with a life expectancy of 177 years and a heart rate of 6 beats per minute, to the hamster with a heart rate of 400 beats per minute that only live about four years.[111]

What intrigue and confusion must have washed over the first mortal soul to discover this thumping object through the chest. "I have been able to hear very plainly the beating of a man's heart," wrote Robert Hooke, a famous English scientist and polymath from the 17th century who was one of the first to describe it. "Who knows, I say, but that it may be possible to discover the motions of the internal parts of the bodies ... by the sound they make."[11] Even prior to Hooke was Dr. William Harvey, who in 1628 published *On the Motion of the Heart and Blood*, noting that "when there is delivery of a quantity of blood from the veins to the arteries, that a pulse takes place, and can be heard within the chest."[112] Yet no formal study of the heart's sounds was undertaken before Laennec and his stethoscope entered the scene. Listening to the heart "conveys to the ear a distinct sound ... and each beat of the arterial pulse corresponds to this double sound," Laennec explained, with the first sound resembling a "pair of bellows" and the other "more dull and prolonged, coinciding with the beat of the pulse."[1]

By this time, the sequence of events in the beating heart was understood quite well. Dr. Harvey knew the atrium contracts and empties into the ventricle after which "the heart raises itself straightway, makes all its fibres tense, contracts the ventricles, and performs a beat," sending the "blood supplied to it ... into the arteries."[112] However, Laennec incorrectly thought the timing was reversed, with the atrium contracting after the ventricle, a belief that was not corrected until 1828, reasserting the sequence Dr. Harvey had explained 200 years prior.[11]

Donkeys, Heart sounds, and Controversy

As word spread about the stethoscope and the science of auscultation, young students from all over Europe flocked to Paris to learn from Laennec and attend his lectures. Two of those students - James Hope and Charles J.B. Williams - would go on to advance the field of cardiac auscultation while bittering their friendship in the process. After graduating college, Hope (Figure 9) followed in Laennec's footsteps, training in Paris at *La Char-*

ite where Laennec worked, adopting his technique of rigorous clinical notes and autopsy correlation. He wrote multiple books documenting his exploration into the human body, most notably was *Diseases of the Heart and Great Vessels*, one of the earliest cardiology textbooks ever written.[11]

At that time, auscultation was still frowned upon by many in the English medical community, something Dr. Hope sought to change. His strategy was judicious, never "argued in favor of auscultation, but allowed facts to speak for themselves." He was always seen at the bedside with a stethoscope and journal in hand, taking very detailed notes, ultimately writing down his presumed diagnosis. Before proceeding to the autopsy, he "publicly placed his book on the table in order that it might be read by all; his diagnosis was invariably correct."[113] Hope had quite the penchant for showmanship, touting the virtues of mediate auscultation in a public demonstration he held in 1838. He gave four novice students a basic lesson in cardiac auscultation, then had them listen to the hearts of various patients with known valvular disease. "Out of sixteen diagnoses which were made," explained one of Hope's students in a letter to the London Medical Gazette, "one alone was partially defective."[114]

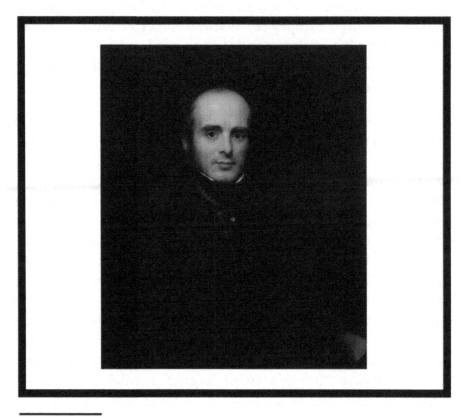

FIGURE 9   Portrait of Dr. James Hope (1801 - 1841), an English physician and pioneer in cardiac auscultation. He wrote one of the first cardiology textbooks and was named "the first cardiologist in the modern sense."

Murmurs from the Valves

In addition to the heart sounds associated with the pulse, Laennec detected other sounds he called "bellows-sounds" due to their auditory resemblance to a fireplace bellow. He thought they sounded like a "continuous murmur, like that of the sea, or that which is produced by the application of a large shell to the ear;" however, he was bewildered by where these sounds were coming from. He looked into the hearts on autopsy and "could discover no organic lesion coinciding constantly with these phenomena," eventually attributing them to spasms in the arteries of the heart.

While murmurs and other heart sounds were known to be correlated with various cardiac diseases, much disagreement was still present over exactly what part of the heart actually made the sounds. In the early 1830s, along with his old friend Charles J.B. Williams, Dr. Hope sought to flesh out this controversy with an experiment to be performed on donkeys in front of a large audience. His first step was to "procure some woorara," a South American arrow poison of which they injected "through an incision into the haunch ... producing insensitivity," enabling them to study the motions and sounds of the donkey's heart for a much longer period.[115] With the audience watching, a hook was inserted into the heart to interfere with each valve while observers listened to the cardiac surface with a stethoscope. This experiment provided the first evidence supporting the valvular origin of heart sounds while turning Hope and Williams against each other in the process, each claiming to have discovered the origin of the heart sounds themselves.[115]

Hope's donkey experiments coupled with his own clinical experience resulted in descriptions of valvular diseases that were truly remarkable for his time. "Diseases of the valves," he explained, "whatever be their nature ... obstruct the orifices of the heart; and this they do, either by contracting the apertures," now known as **stenosis** of the valves, or in *regurgitation* "by encumbering the valves in such a manner as to prevent them from opening and closing with suitable accuracy and facility." And he knew that turbulent blood flow through these diseased valves was the cause of the heart murmurs heard through the stethoscope.[18]

Hope correctly described the murmur caused by *aortic valve stenosis* as being "heard during ventricular contraction (i.e. with the first sound) on the sternum ... Its pitch or key is usually that of a whispered *r*." He was also able to accurately describe *aortic regurgitation* as a murmur that "accompanies the second sound ... always imparting to it the bellows-murmur ... like whispering the word *awe* during inspiration." He thought *mitral regurgitation* had a low key, "more like whispering *who*," while the *mitral stenosis* murmur "attends the ventricular diastole and second sound", and was "always very feeble." His precise descriptions of murmurs were in stark contrast to Laennec's, who could not pinpoint their cause. According to Hope, this was due to Laennec's attribution of the second heart sound to the atrium, a mistake that "perplexed him in referring murmurs to their true source."

In the decades that followed, our understanding of cardiac auscultation went through multiple refinements. From influential physicians like Drs. Austin Flint, Graham Steell or W. Proctor Harvey, to the development of recorded phonocardiography that helped clinicians better understand the hemodynamic properties of heart murmurs.[116] This brought auscultation to its pinnacle in cardiac diagnostics, when a physician with a stethoscope and a pair of highly trained ears was the only practical bedside method of diagnosing cardiac disease.

Auscultation and Accuracy

The ability of a stethoscope-wielding clinician to diagnose valvular disease through auscultation varies greatly by many factors, such as the experience and abilities of the listener, the noise of the ambient environment, or the type and severity of the valvular pathology. A severe aortic stenosis murmur in a cardiologist's quiet office, for example, is far simpler to detect than a low-frequency diastolic murmur in a busy emergency department.

In 1870, Dr. Austin Flint confidently proclaimed that "the absence of a murmur ... warrants the conclusion that the lesions do not exist, the probability of error being exceedingly small."[117] Yet despite such rhetoric that accompanied "the golden age" of stethoscopic cardiac diagnostics, studies evaluating the sensitivity and specificity of auscultation, whether by medical trainees or experienced cardiologists, are less than golden. For example, in a study of medical residents at Duke University using a cardiac sound simulator, the residents correctly identified mitral regurgitation only 52% of the time, mitral stenosis only 37% of the time, and aortic regurgitation 54% of the time.[118] A 1997 study similarly found that internal medicine and family medicine residents who were asked to identify 12 common cardiac abnormalities from patient recordings "were incorrect 4 of 5 times, improved little with a year of training, and were not more accurate than a group of medical students."[119] Such results could be chalked up to poor training or lack of experience were they not also seen in studies of real patients being assessed by board-certified cardiologists.

The very notion that valvular disease can be detected at all with auscultation is based most fundamentally on the assumption that most, if not all, clinically significant valvular pathologies make a sound that is audible to the human ear. Of course, if they are present but don't make a sound, a stethoscope by definition could not detect them. With the advent of echocardiography, this underlying assumption has been tested in various capacities throughout the medical literature.

For example, in a study of regurgitation murmurs in a hospital setting, internal medicine residents and cardiologists listened to the hearts of 294 patients and their physical exam findings were compared to the results of an echocardiogram. The cardiologists had excellent specificity to rule in regurgitant valves when a murmur was detected, yet they missed 70% of mitral regurgitation cases, 88% of the tricuspid regurgitation cases, and 63% of aortic regurgitation cases that were present on the echocardiograms. This led the author to conclude that "the sensitivity of auscultation, overall, was extremely low," and that contrary to Dr. Flint's belief that the absence of an audible murmur rules out disease, "our data suggest that there is a high prevalence of 'silent' murmurs. Consequently, when it is important to know whether regurgitation is present, auscultation alone, even if negative, will not suffice."[120] Very similar results were found in another study of regurgitant murmurs assessed by a cardiologist where an audible murmur was only heard in 56% of patients with mitral regurgitation, 61% of patients with aortic regurgitation, and 28% in patients with tricuspid regurgitation.[121]

In a more recent study from 2000, a group of cardiologists examined 100 patients and again compared their results to an echocardiogram. In this group, the cardiologists with a stethoscope were able to detect isolated mitral regurgitation in 88% of patients who had it and aortic stenosis in 71%. 27% of moderate-to-severe aortic stenosis cases and 79% of aortic regurgitation lesions were missed, and only half of the patients with both aortic and mitral valve disease were correctly diagnosed. "Although the cardiac examination remains the first-line tool of every clinician," they concluded, "physicians should be aware of these limitations."[122]

This poor ability to detect significant valvular disease with auscultation is not unique to the United States. Physicians in Copenhagen, for example, listened to 2,907 patients admitted to the hospital and correctly detected a murmur in patients with valvular heart disease with only 52% sensitivity but an impressive 93% specificity.[123] In the United Kingdom, 251 patients were screened by experienced primary care physicians and cardiologists with a stethoscope in another study. Only 44% of the moderate-to-severe valvular pathologies were detected by the primary care physicians with only 69% specificity, while only 31% were detected by the cardiologists with 81% specificity.[124] Finally, in a Swiss study of patients with known valvular heart diseases from 2010, blinded cardiologists with a stethoscope only diagnosed 76% of patients of correctly, while the internists were only correct 64% of the time.[125]

The Plausible vs the Possible

While the diagnostic accuracy varies within the literature, the hypothesis that all clinically important valvular diseases emit stethoscope-detectable sounds is not supported by the majority of studies. This consistently poor sensitivity means that even in the hands of experienced cardiologists, the absence of a murmur does not rule out valvular disease, and in the hands of anyone else, such findings are even less fruitful. On the other hand, many studies do show relatively high specificity of isolated aortic stenosis or mitral regurgitation murmurs suggesting that if such a murmur is heard - especially by a cardiologist - there is a good chance it is a result of real valvular disease. Therefore, while listening for murmurs to detect all significant valvular disease is plausible, in practice the data do not support most clinicians' ability to adequately do so. Or as Dutch cardiologist and POCUS pioneer Dr. Roelandt put it: "The performance of the traditional physical examination has been evaluated in several studies, indicating that 30% major and 65% minor pathologies are missed. Correct identification of heart sounds and murmurs ranged between 20 and 50% ... Would these results pass the current tests applied in clinical trials for reliability?"[126]

Just as with lung auscultation from Part I, the real question regarding the utility of cardiac auscultation though, is *compared to what?* Compared to not listening at all, or to immediate auscultation with the ear flush against the chest it is certainly better. But in the *POCUS Era*, we must also compare these findings to what can now be achieved with appropriate training and a pocket-sized ultrasound device.

CHAPTER 11: CARDIAC ULTRASOUND ORIGINS

"All around us technology is moving at a breathtaking pace and influencing our daily lives in ways unimaginable just a few years ago. Yet we walk around with the stethoscope in our pockets or around our necks! It is time that we put aside this 200-year-old technology and embrace the modern world. Otherwise we will look like dinosaurs!"

DR. SANJIV KAUL, CARDIOLOGIST, OREGON HEALTH
AND SCIENCE UNIVERSITY, 2014

Situated in the southwest tip of Sweden sits the city of Lund, where two cardiac surgeons - Drs. Helge Wulff and Phillip Sandblom - were operating on patients with severe mitral stenosis in the 1940s. Once the chest was opened and the mitral valve revealed, the surgeons would dilate the narrowed valve with their fingers, causing many patients to improve. However, some patients also had a component of *mitral regurgitation*, a leaking of the valve that worsened with this finger dilation.[127] This created an opportunity for Dr. Inge Edler, a physician from Malmö who moved to Lund to become the director of this cardiovascular lab at the University Hospital, responsible for pre-operative cardiac evaluations.[128] He was tasked with determining which patients had pure mitral stenosis and would benefit from surgery, yet there was no good method for identifying these patients at the time.

Edler was an amateur magician, an avid bicycle acrobatist till the age of 75, and an overall curious man with varied interests. As scientists around the world were looking to repurpose wartime technologies for other uses after World War II,[129] Edler hypothesized that one of those technologies, sound navigation and ranging or SONAR, could help with his clinical dilemma. He consulted with his clinic nurse who was married to a physicist, and her husband, in turn, thought of a friend who may be able to help: a man named Hellmuth Hertz.[130]

Hertz came from a distinguished pedigree of physicists, with his father winning the Nobel Prize in Physics. Not to mention his uncle, Heinrich Hertz, the same Heinrich Hertz that lent his name to the unit of frequency. Dr. Edler presented his idea of using sonar-based ultrasound to study the heart to Hertz who was intrigued, and thought ultrasound may work. In 1953, they went to a shipyard nearby that had an ultrasound machine. Hertz placed the probe on his chest and a moving signal appeared. The first cardiac ultrasound, he wondered? By pure luck, this machine happened to have a transducer with the correct wavelength to see the heart. If it were lower or higher, they may not have detected anything.

To understand exactly what he was seeing on this new ultrasound device, Edler would conduct clever yet morbid sonographic exams on patients near death. He marked the direction of the ultrasound beam on the patient's chest, and when they passed away, he passed an ice pick through the chest wall in the direction taken by the ultrasound beam. Then on autopsy, he traced where in the heart the ice pick had pierced and compared that distance to the distance of the ultrasound signal on the screen. He figured out that the tip of the ice pick had entered through the mitral valve, which was causing the signal in question, and was eventually able to identify the signal a stenotic mitral valve made compared to a regurgitant one.

Just as with Drs. Laennec and Lichtenstein, there was a cold reception for Edler and Hertz's discovery. They presented their methods to Dr. Andre F. Cournand, a physician who received the Nobel prize for his contributions to cardiac catheterization, who was not impressed. They also showed it to President Dwight D. Eisenhower's cardiologist Paul Dudley White who politely dismissed it as unimportant. Likewise, they could not get funding from the Swedish Board of Technical Development, because they believed it lacked medical or commercial interest.

These rejections proved insurmountable, and Edler's interest in ultrasound fizzled as his technique for identifying mitral stenosis turned out to not be very precise and was eventually discredited.[131] Fortunately for the future of cardiac diagnostics, a very similar story was unfolding in the United States, led by a young cardiologist named Harvey Feigenbaum.

Feigenbaum's Discovery

Like every day at work, Dr. Harvey Feigenbaum was eating lunch in his office when he came across an advertisement in a random journal on his desk. The ad was from a company named *BioSonar,* promoting a product that they claimed could measure heart volumes with ultrasound. It was an idea that intrigued Feigenbaum since he was struggling with the concept of measuring heart volumes during cardiac catheterizations at the time. He called the number on the advertisement and found out they'd be showing their new device at the upcoming *American Heart Association* meeting in 1963. Feigenbaum attended that meeting and beelined to the *BioSonar* booth. He asked the person working there how to use their device to measure cardiac volumes, to which the *BioSonar* representative responded: "What are cardiac volumes?"[132]

It turned out the advertisement Feigenbaum saw was quite misleading since the machine actually used ultrasound to detect the midline of the brain, not volumes of the heart. Confused as to why such a machine was at a cardiology conference, Feigenbaum placed the machine's probe on his chest and immediately saw a moving spike. "It was obviously related to my heart ... the way it was moving, the timing of it, location of it. It had to be coming from the back wall of my heart."[129] Excited about his discovery, Feigenbaum wondered if it could detect a pericardial effusion.

Back at the hospital, he borrowed a similar machine from the neurology department and began examining patients with it, seeing the same, singular moving echo signal from the heart. He found a patient with a known pericardial effusion and placed it on their chest. "Just as I predicted, instead of one signal that was moving, I saw 2 signals. One was moving and the other was stationary, and the space between the two had to be the effusion."

He called Dr. John Waldhausen, a cardiac surgeon who had an animal laboratory, and they set up a study in dogs to see if these findings could be reproduced. "We injected saline into the pericardial space and the singular signal divided into 2, one moving and one stationary. We took the fluid out and the signals or echoes came back together. We repeated this routine in 5 consecutive dogs and that was it. It happened every time." They published a paper titled *Ultrasound Diagnosis of Pericardial Effusion*[133] in 1965 documenting their findings, but it largely fell on deaf ears. "By the time that I came up with ultrasound, they decided it was garbage," Feigenbaum later recalled.[134] "The skepticism was overwhelming. I had the misfortune to follow ballistocardiography (a technique based on recording the effect of heart contraction on the body as recorded on a motion-sensitive table), which was a disaster. Skeptics said: here we go again."

Dr. W. Proctor Harvey, a famous cardiologist at Georgetown University who ran the largest and most competitive cardiology fellowship at the time "completely refused to accept echocardiography," and was "completely wedded to the physical examination with auscultation." Likewise, the editor of the *American Heart Journal*, a premier cardiology journal at the time, declined to publish on echocardiography.

Even the manufacturer of the ultrasound machine Feigenbaum was using at the time, *Smith-Kline*, was going to give up as well if it wasn't for one man at the company named Tom Davis. He believed in Feigenbaum's work and invited him to one of their marketing meetings in 1965. Feigenbaum gave a presentation arguing that "cardiac ultrasound would be a major diagnostic tool because we are "seeing the heart." Those signals were coming from the heart! How can that not be important!?"

Dr. Edler had faced much of the same pushback and spent almost 10 years working on ultrasound but eventually gave up. "The main difference between us was that I was dead set on cardiac ultrasound and he wasn't," Feigenbaum explained. "Inge was a wonderful human being. We spent a lot of time together both in Europe and the United States," but his work with echo was short-lived, and his main findings turned out to not be very useful. Despite this fact, according to Feigenbaum, his European colleagues tended to glorify Edler's contributions and downplay his, as evidenced by the fact that the European Society of Echocardiology (now called Cardiovascular Imaging) didn't get around to making him an honorary member until 2014.[131]

Feigenbaum's passion and determination convinced *Smith-Kline* to continue making their device, enabling him to continue his work in developing the field. His work in ultrasound eventually earned him the title of "the father of echocardiography," revolutionizing the field of cardiac diagnostics forever (Figure 10).

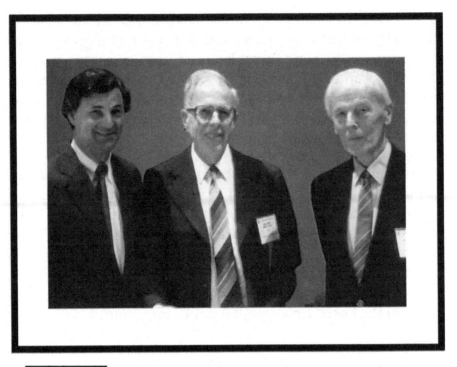

FIGURE 10   Harvey Feigenbaum (left), Helmuth Hertz (center) and Inge
Edler in 1988 at a meeting in Indianapolis celebrating Dr.
Feigenbaum's 25th anniversary working with echocardiography.

Used with permission from Dr. Feigenbaum

CHAPTER 12: CARDIAC POINT-OF-CARE ULTRASOUND

"Future generations of doctors will find it hard to believe that, in 2013, many clinicians were still relying on the vague findings of a 200-year-old traditional physical examination and were compromising clinical efficacy when direct information was available from point-of-care echocardiography. History will undoubtedly show that point-of-care echocardiography was the beginning of a 'new glorious age' of the physical examination."

DR. JOS ROELANDT, CARDIOLOGIST & POCUS PIONEER,
2013

In its most basic sense, the physical exam is a method of inferring the state of health of the internal organs. In the *Before POCUS era*, this is accomplished through auscultation, inspection, palpation, and percussion. These techniques complement the taking of a detailed history, designed to flesh out uncertainties arising from the patient's subjective report. However, such methods are often so imprecise that they do little to reduce uncertainty or narrow our differential diagnosis at all.

As the field of echocardiography was developing among cardiologists, the visual study of the heart was clearly offering more detailed and accurate information than auscultation could. With rapid advancements improving ultrasound technology and miniaturizing the hardware it required, various physicians envisioned pocket-sized devices that could view the heart as routinely as we listen to it. Dr. Jos Roelandt was one such cardiologist from the Netherlands who integrated POCUS into his physical exams as early as 1978. He and his colleagues "constructed a hand-held battery-powered ultrasound imager" they named "the ultrasound stethoscope," that he used in his patient examinations. He was able to diagnose pericardial effusions, estimate cardiac chamber size, and look for valvular disease.[126]

He recognized the limitations of our physical exam to detect things like early heart failure or silent valvular disease that are "a challenge to the most experienced clinician or even impossible, while they are rapidly diagnosed by echo." Why then, he wondered in an opinion piece he wrote in 2013, "should we rely on indirect information and secondary acoustic events when we actually can see what is wrong with the heart and its structures?"

Nowhere is this more evident than with the diagnosis of *heart failure with a reduced ejection fraction*. Since the days of Drs. Laennec and Hope, the signs and symptoms of congestive heart failure and its downstream ramifications have been well understood. Laennec knew there was a "habitually swelled state of the veins," and Dr. Hope understood that fluid backs up into the lungs and into the rest of the body through "a series of striking phenomena," starting with lower extremity swelling that "gradually ascends, and under the name of anasarca, may eventually attain the utmost degree over the whole surface of the body."[18] However, since these signs or symptoms are not specific to congestive heart failure, the direct diagnosis of a reduced ejection fraction has remained elusive.

In the *Before POCUS era*, listening for a **third heart sound**, or *S3*, is another sign that has been employed toward this evasive diagnosis. It was initially described by French physician Dr. Pierre

Potain in 1847 as "three sounds, namely: two normal sounds of the heart and a superadded sound ... this is the bruit de galop,"[135] becoming the subject of much scientific inquiry ever since. This third heart sound is considered normal when heard in younger patients, but after 40 years of age it is pathologic, a sign that is quite specific though not very sensitive. The diagnostic accuracies vary wildly in the literature, with sensitivities of 26-69%,[136,137] while a review in the *Journal of the American Medical Association* placed the sensitivity and specificity at 13% and 99% respectively.[138]

In more recent studies, however, this third heart sound was less specific. For example, in a study of 580 patients from 2001, it was only 45% sensitive and 87% specific for patients with congestive heart failure.[136] Likewise, in a study of cardiologists' auscultation abilities, the detection of an S3 was 68% sensitive and 73% specific for heart failure,[137] while in a 2014 study of over 1300 patients with congestive heart failure and reduced ejection fraction, cardiologists only heard an S3 in 15% of them.[139] In addition to its poor accuracy, the ability to detect a third heart sound is confounded by the fact that it is a very low-frequency sound and therefore difficult to confidently hear,[116] and shows poor agreement regarding its existence when different physicians examine the same patient.[140,141]

Seeing is Believing

This prospect of diagnosing congestive heart failure with certainty at the bedside would dramatically improve our physical examination and expedite care, instead of relying on an echocardiogram which can take hours to weeks depending on the clinical setting. In the *POCUS Era*, we do not need to rely on "secondary acoustic events" as there are much more precise methods for determining if the patient has a reduced ejection fraction. By employing a simplified, qualitative method borrowed from echocardiography, the ejection fraction can be estimated with cardiac POCUS as normal, reduced, or severely reduced. This "eyeball method" can be accurately achieved by non cardiologists,[142-147] and improve the diagnostic accuracy in a patient with congestive heart failure. Such results were evident in a study of medical students and residents from 2012, for example. Using just signs and symptoms of congestive heart failure acquired through a traditional physical exam, they detected a reduced ejection fraction with 25% sensitivity and 84% specificity. However, with the addition of cardiac POCUS and only two hours of training these figures rose to 74% and 93.6% respectively.[148]

The capability of our physical exam to diagnose cardiovascular disease has been scrutinized in various *stethoscope-versus-POCUS* studies, invariably showing improved diagnostic accuracy with POCUS. In a 2001 study out of the University of Chicago, cardiologists with a stethoscope failed to detect 59% of known cardiac pathologies compared to the POCUS group who missed 29%. If only major cardiovascular findings were considered, cardiologists missed 43% while the POCUS group missed only 21%.[149] With the stethoscope, they missed 57% of mitral regurgitation murmurs and 76% of tricuspid regurgitation murmurs. They did well with aortic stenosis, detecting 88%, however they were particularly bad with diastolic murmurs, only detecting 26%. Two-thirds of the cardiologists could not identify patients with reduced ejection fraction with physical exam alone, while only 23% were missed with POCUS. Overall the diagnostic accuracy with POCUS was superior to the stethoscope in almost every cardiac pathology, and the authors concluded that although "cardiac auscultation has excellent specificity, the sensitivity of this technique in the current era is remarkably low."[149]

In a more recent study with modernized, pocket-sized ultrasound devices, the physical exams performed by 17 different cardiologists with a stethoscope were compared to the results with cardiac POCUS. Overall, the cardiologists detected only 47% of all abnormalities while 82% were detected with POCUS. The bedside ultrasound diagnosed 71% of moderate-to-severe valvular diseases compared to 31% in the physical exam group. 96% of patients with reduced ejection fraction were accurately diagnosed with POCUS compared to 35% with the exam and stethoscope (Table 5).[150] The handheld ultrasound group was universally superior to the physical examination group, leading the authors to declare that "a physician could have an all-purpose tool in his or her pocket" that provides "timely and more accurate diagnosis than physical examination for the majority of common cardiovascular abnormalities." It is a bedside diagnostic tool "that would be more in keeping with the 21st century than the stethoscope, a 200-year-old technology whose time should be over."[151]

ECHO FINDING	POCUS % CORRECT	PHYSICAL EXAM % CORRECT	% IMPROVEMENT WITH POCUS
Normal Ejection Fraction	89%	58%	31%
Reduced Ejection Fraction	96%	35%	61%
Normal Right Ventricle Function	94%	57%	37%
Abnormal Right Ventricle Function	68%	21%	47%
Mild or Absent Valve Disease	94%	91%	3.5%
Moderate-Severe Valve Disease	71%	31%	39%

TABLE 5   DIAGNOSING CARDIAC DISEASE

Diagnostic accuracy of POCUS compared to traditional physical exam by cardiologists and percent improvement with POCUS. Adapted from study of 250 patients. Mehta et al 2014.

Similar improvement to the physical exam with POCUS has been confirmed by numerous similar studies,[148,152–159] solidifying cardiac POCUS as a more accurate and effective method for diagnosing cardiac disease at the bedside.

Redefining "Physical Exam"

In the *POCUS Era*, murmurs can be seen, not just heard. A reduced ejection fraction is detected, not inferred, and the presence of a pericardial effusion is confirmed or denied, not hypothesized. In a 200 year span, the weeks-long, meticulous auscultation-to-autopsy strategy Laennec or Hope had to employ to understand cardiac disease can now be achieved with far greater accuracy in just a few minutes, with a dollop of gel and a well-positioned ultrasound probe. What excitement and disbelief might strike Dr. Hope today were he able to look inside his patients while still alive and see a diseased heart, beating in real-time; and what disgust or bewilderment he may feel toward those who scoff at such potential, blinded by their dogmatic defense of a 200-year-old tool. With multiple pocket-sized, increasingly affordable ultrasound probes on the market, it is time to expand the classical limitations of what exactly a 'physical exam' is and incorporate cardiac POCUS, building upon what Dr. Roelandt advocated more than four decades ago.

CHAPTER 13: INTERNAL JUGULAR VEIN & THE VOLUME EXAM

"From the dilation of the right auricle and ventricle there are two especially important results, for it is they above all that bring about the alternating dilation of the jugulars."

DR. GIOVANNI LANCISI, ON THE MOTION OF THE
HEART AND ON ANEURYSMS, 1728

Of all the physical exam skills a clinician learns throughout their training, perhaps the examination of the jugular vein is the most iconic. It entails visually inspecting the lateral portion of a patient's neck, looking for the top of the blood column in the ***internal jugular vein***, and estimating the distance from there down to the heart. It was first described in 1930 by Sir Thomas Lewis,[160] a famed British cardiologist equipped with a delightfully bushy mustache. Physicians as far back as Dr. Giovanni Lancisi in the early 18th century had already known that veins engorge in congestive heart failure;[161] however, Lewis was one of the first to qualitatively measure the degree of distension.

He explained that congestive heart failure manifests itself "first in breathlessness, and continuing in its natural development to profound engagement of the venous system." These symptoms often have an insidious onset, starting with shortness of breath with exercise and progressing ultimately to shortness of breath at rest. It is during this progression, he explained, when the signs of engorged veins first appear, which is why he felt every medical student "should make a full study of them."

Calculating the Jugular Venous Pressure (JVP)

In a semi-upright position, the internal jugular vein is partially filled with blood and collapses above the level that blood reaches up to.[162] It functions to drain deoxygenated blood into the right heart, via two even larger vessels: the subclavian vein and the superior vena cava. For simplicity's sake, it can be thought of as a graduated cylinder, with the right atrium as its base and the jugular vein as its walls. The top of the blood column that fills the internal jugular vein in this simplified model is called the *meniscus*, which corresponds to the *jugular venous pulsation* since the top of the blood column is where the pulsations are most prominent. Therefore, the vertical distance from this meniscus down to the center of the right atrium is equal to the *jugular venous pressure*, which corresponds to the *right atrial pressure* (Figure 11).

The internal jugular vein is made up of two important segments: the *obscured portion* below the clavicle, and the remaining *visible portion* above the clavicle up to the patient's jaw. In a healthy person with normal right atrial pressures, the meniscus does not reach the *visible portion* of the internal jugular vein, and therefore the vein is fully collapsed above the clavicle and cannot be seen. As the patient becomes more "congested," Lewis explained, the veins engorge and the pressure rises, displacing this meniscus previously obscured below the clavicle upwards toward the jawline where it can be seen through the skin of the neck in the *visible portion* of the internal jugular vein.

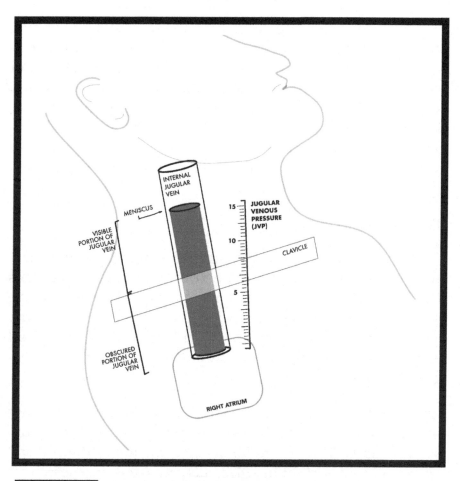

FIGURE 11 Simplified schematic of the internal jugular vein and right atrium. The classical JVP exam looks for the meniscus in the visible portion of the vein. The vertical distance from this point down to the right atrium is used to estimate the jugular venous pressure, which should correlate with the right atrial pressure.

This pressure could be measured *directly* with an invasive right heart catheterization procedure; however, this is not possible at the patient's bedside. Instead, as Lewis demonstrated, since the vein is often visible through the skin, the right atrial pressure can be *indirectly* estimated by measuring the height of the blood column in the internal jugular vein.

Once the meniscus on the neck has been identified, the *vertical distance* from this point down to the sternum is recorded, estimating the height of the blood column in the *visible portion* of the vein. This is then added to the distance from the sternum down to the right atrium (corresponding to the *obscured portion* of the vein), which is classically assumed to be five centimeters.[163] Adding those together, a jugular venous pressure over nine centimeters of water is considered abnormally high.[164]

"JVP Not Appreciated"

The importance of accurately measuring jugular venous pressure (JVP) stems from the diametrically opposed treatments that low and high pressures require. As Dr. Lewis explained, the proper use of this jugular exam "will save a very large number of serious diagnostic blunders," since high pressures and fluid excess calls for diuretics, while low pressure and fluid dearth necessitates the opposite.

Yet while this concept is well understood and accepted, it is not uncommon to see a cardiologist, a nephrologist, and a hospitalist come up with wildly different assessments of the JVP and overall fluid assessment in a given patient. Some may perceive it to be elevated and recommend diuretics, while others may not detect it at all and recommend IV fluids. *How can this be?*

When a clinician does not detect an elevated jugular venous pressure, they often document this as "JVP not appreciated," but what exactly does "not appreciated" mean? Is the patient overweight and the vein cannot be visualized? Or is the pressure in the venous system low enough that the JVP does not rise above the clavicle to be seen? Or is the clinician not experienced and does not see the JVP due to his or her own negligence? Unfortunately, our current methods don't offer enough accuracy to answer these questions.

In 1974, internal medicine physicians at Northwestern University studied whether the *method of Lewis* correlated with the right atrial pressure, also known as the **central venous pressure (CVP)**. They examined the external and internal jugular veins and compared them to the gold standard values obtained from a CVP catheter, which sits in the venous system just outside the right atrium and provides real-time pressure readings. While their measurements from the **external jugular vein** correlated with CVP, only half of those readings were within 2 centimeters of the actual value. Interestingly, when trying to do the same correlation with the **internal jugular vein** used in the **method of Lewis**, they found that "the internal jugular veins were frequently difficult to visualize," and therefore the sample was too small to analyze. To obtain a 90 percent concordance between the external jugular vein estimate and the CVP catheter, they explained, "an error of up to 4 cm had to be allowed. Moreover, large discrepancies were noted in individual cases," concluding that the central venous pressure "cannot be reliably estimated by inspection of the jugular veins."[165]

In another study from 1983 published in the *New England Journal of Medicine*,[166] clinicians tried to estimate right atrial pressure in 56 critically ill patients, comparing their results to the gold standard right heart catheterization measurements. While there was a modest correlation between the JVP estimation and the right atrial pressure, the results were "better than random; however, the percentage of accurate predictions was quite low," at about 42%. A clinical exam of critically ill patients they noted, "does not provide enough information to assess hemodynamic status accurately." Similar results were seen in two other studies of ICU patients,[167,168] as well as in a study of medical residents assessing the jugular vein from 2007. They were only able to visualize the meniscus in 37% of patients who had it in the visible portion of the vein and were particularly poor at correctly detecting elevated pressures, with only 14% sensitivity.[152]

Such results are analogous to those from a group of intensive care physicians who underwent a JVP assessment teaching session prior to the start of another study. Despite this added educational piece, the clinical JVP assessment for determining high right atrial pressure was limited, with a sensitivity of 43% and a specificity of 67%.[169] Even with experienced cardiologists, the sensitivity and specificity of an elevated JVP exam to predict high right atrial pressure was 65% and 85% respectively when compared to pressures measured with a right heart catheterization.[170] These limitations to the visual assessment of jugular venous pressure were summarized in a review article out of the University of Washington, arguing that most studies of JVP exams were inaccurate and unreliable, concluding that not much progress has been made since Sir Thomas Lewis first took a shot at it in the early 1930s.[171]

Limitations to the Method of Lewis

The hard truth is that no matter how good the clinician, no matter how detail-oriented or experienced, there are two rules of the JVP that cannot be overcome:

1. The meniscus or jugular venous pulsation that cannot be seen cannot be evaluated
2. The JVP measurement relying on assumptions will invariably fail

JVP Not Visible

If the jugular venous pulsations are not visualized, then one of four things are true:

1. It is present and visible but the clinician did not detect it
2. The pressure is low enough in the jugular vein that the meniscus is below the clavicle and cannot be seen
3. The pressure is so high that the meniscus resides above the jawline and the pulsations are not present in the neck
4. The patient's anatomy does not allow for it to be visualized.

Complicating the JVP assessment further may be a patient's thick neck or a large beard, or the fact that - in the United States at least - over 70% of patients are overweight or obese.[172] In these patients, the meniscus may literally be invisible and therefore the *method of Lewis* simply cannot be used.

Or maybe a pulsation is seen in the neck but it is not entirely clear whether it is the JVP or the carotid artery sitting next door to it. It is also possible the clinician was correct when saying it was "not appreciated" if the jugular venous pressure is in fact normal. Ultimately this creates a certainty-free zone leading to low confidence in our decision making.

Assumptions Lead to Failure

Sir Thomas Lewis's method has stood the test of time for providing a rough, qualitative estimate of right atrial pressure. However, researchers have consistently come up short when attempting to quantify it with an actual pressure value. These failures are due in part to the assumption that the distance from the sternum down to the right atrium (here on referred to as **right atrial depth**), corresponding to the *obscured portion* of the vein, is 5 centimeters when in fact it often is not.

This chosen distance originated from a 1946 study in which they snaked a urinary catheter with a pressure sensor on it up through the arm veins and into the right atrium to measure the right atrial pressures in real-time.[173] They wanted to choose a reference point that passes "somewhere through the heart itself and at the same time bear a reasonably constant relationship to an external landmark," such as the top of the sternum. With the patient lying flat on their back, the right atrial depth was measured from a chest X-ray to be around 5.8 cm, yet for "the sake of simplicity ... it has been decided to take the conventional venous pressure reference level of 5 cm" below the sternum. However, a more recent study of thoracic CT scans suggests the actual right atrial depth is nearly double that at 9 centimeters, and that using the standard 5 centimeter assumption incorrectly estimates the right atrial depth 71% of the time.[174] This right atrial depth also varies significantly based on the patient's position and body size. As the head of the bed is raised and the angle increases from zero, another study using CT scans found that the median distance is about 8.8 centimeters at 30 degrees and 9.9 centimeters at 45 degrees, with enormous variation from 5 to 15 centimeters depending on the patient's age, body size, and smoking status.[175] While the median is useful in the aggregate, in each patient the degree of variation is so large that an assumption may be off by as much at 10 centimeters of water. Therefore, for any method to be successful, it must measure this distance in each patient, an impractical feat without the use of ultrasound.

CHAPTER 14: JVP ALWAYS APPRECIATED

"His jugular arteries, enlarged to the size of the thumb, looked like the aorta itself ... they had pulsated violently, and appeared like two long aneurisms. These symptoms had led to trying the effects of arteriotomy in the temples, but with no relief. In the dead body I found the heart and aorta so much gorged and distended with blood, that the cavities of the ventricles equalled those of a bullock's heart in size."

DR. WILLIAM HARVEY, 1578 - 1657

The inability to measure **right atrial depth** coupled with the imprecise visualization of the meniscus renders the method of Lewis impossible to perform accurately in many patients. However, both of these limitations can be elegantly overcome using ultrasound. With POCUS, the jugular vein is *always appreciated*, since it sits so close to the skin and is easily identified regardless of the patient's neck size or BMI. It can be viewed **longitudinally**, with the probe parallel to the vein in the head-to-toe axis of the body, or in the **transverse** view, with the probe sitting perpendicular to the vein in the left-to-right axis.

As discussed previously, with a patient sitting upright at 90 degrees, the vein is partially filled, though usually not enough to displace the meniscus into the visible portion of the vein, unless the right atrial pressure is very high. As the angle of the bed reduces and the patient moves toward being supine, the blood will spread towards the head and fill the vein, just as a partially filled bottle of cabernet when placed on its side. This brings the meniscus, or top of the blood column, above the clavicle and into view of the ultrasound probe. In the head-to-toe (longitudinal) axis, this point looks like the top of a wine bottle,[176] from here on referred to as the *wine bottle sign*. This is the sonographic manifestation of the meniscus, a sight that would probably bring joy to Sir Thomas Lewis were he alive today (Figure 12).

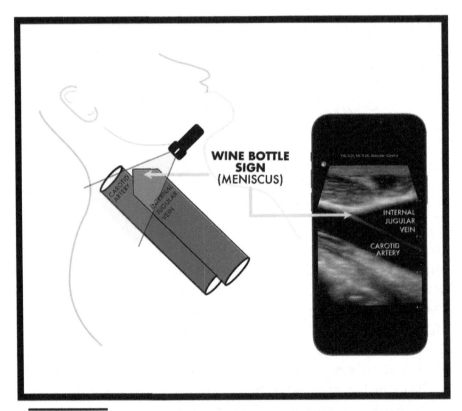

FIGURE 12   Longitudinal view of the internal jugular vein and wine bottle sign. The collapse point (meniscus) takes a triangular shape. This is the sonographic manifestation of the jugular venous pulsations classically visualized on the neck.

Above this wine bottle sign, the vein will collapse, while below the wine bottle sign will be a rounded vein filled with blood. In an abnormally dilated vein (i.e. with *jugular venous distention* or *JVD*) minimal or absent pulsations will be present.

Valsalva and JVD

When the patient reaches zero degrees and is lying flat on their back, the meniscus is no longer present and the vein has reached its maximally engorged state, the extent to which varies by the amount of blood present. In a patient with severe heart failure who has a large amount of excess fluid accumulation, the jugular vein diameter will be very large, while in a healthy patient, it will only partially engorge. The maximum diameter a jugular vein can mount may be determined by asking the patient to bear down as if they are having a bowel movement, called the *Valsalva maneuver*. This forced expiration compresses the heart and blood vessels inside the thorax, displacing the blood into the jugular vein, causing it to dilate 20-30% in patients with normal right atrial pressure.[177] Therefore, in a patient with *jugular venous distention* and elevated right atrial pressure, performing the Valsalva maneuver should cause a smaller increase in the diameter since it is already abnormally distended at rest.

Cardiologists at the Pittsburgh School of Medicine used this physiological fact to categorize the jugular venous pressure as high (greater than or equal to 12 mmHg) or low if 11mmHg or less (Figure 13). They found that if the increase in the cross-sectional area of the internal jugular vein was *less than* 17%, this predicted an elevated right atrial pressure with 90% sensitivity and 74% specificity, while if it increased *more than* 17%, it "all but rules out high right atrial pressure ... with a 94% negative predictive value."[178]

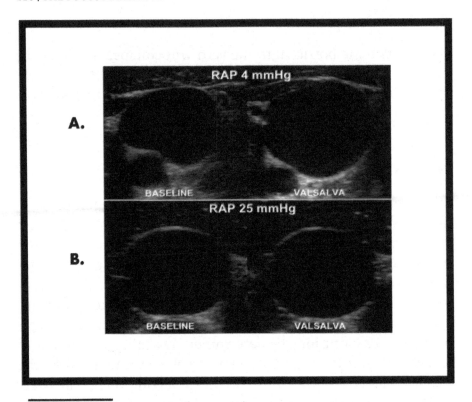

FIGURE 13   **A.** Cross section of normal jugular vein in supine patient with right atrial pressure of 4 mmHg (left) and after valsalva (right)

B. Cross section of distended jugular vein with very elevated right atrial pressure (left) and almost no change during valsalva (right)

Adapted from Simon et al 2010 with permission

The relative distention of the internal jugular vein at rest was also shown to relate to an elevated right atrial pressure in a study of emergency room patients. A jugular vein diameter under 8 millimeters corresponded to a right atrial pressure of less than 10 centimeters of water, while a vein diameter over 11 millimeters was seen with right atrial pressure greater than 10.[179] In both of these studies, the jugular vein was visualized in every patient, regardless of body size or neck anatomy.

Other researchers have attempted a *sonographic method of Lewis*, using ultrasound to identify the meniscus and measure down to the sternum in the *visual portion* of the jugular vein, while still relying on the 5-centimeter assumption for right atrial depth. The wine bottle sign was successfully detected with ultrasound in all jugular veins visualized, even when the standard exam was unsuccessful. However, both studies found that the JVP under-estimated the actual right atrial pressure,[180,181] findings that may be explained simply by the fact that the average right atrial depth is actually nine centimeters not five.[174,175]

Right Heart Catheterizations & Right Atrial Depth

When clinical exams are difficult in certain patients, ultimately the determination of right atrial pressure and overall volume status must be obtained through a right heart catheterization to measure the pressures directly. In this procedure, a catheter is maneuvered through the veins into the right atrium where the pressure is recorded. It is then advanced through the tricuspid valve into the right ventricle and past the pulmonic valve into the pulmonary artery, swimming alongside the deoxygenated blood going towards the lungs. The catheter can make it towards the end of the pulmonary artery, but it can't go into the lung circulation. At this point, the catheter is "wedged" at the end of the pulmonary artery with an inflatable balloon obstructing blood flow temporarily. This technique allows for the catheter to measure the pressure on the other side of the balloon, called the *pulmonary capillary wedge pressure* (or just *wedge pressure* for short). This wedge pressure is often a good surrogate for the pressures in the left side of the heart.

This procedure allows for multiple important, accurate meas-urements of cardiac function such as pulmonary artery pres-sures or right atrial pressures. Cardiac catheterizations are extremely safe; however, even in hospitals performing large numbers each year, there is still about a 1% chance of complica-tions such as clot formation, stroke, bleeding, or vascular compromise related to the procedure, and about a 0.05% chance of death.[182,183] Therefore, if determination of the right atrial pressure and volume status is the clinical question, very accurate sonographic measurements could theoretically replace the need for right heart catheterizations in certain situations and reduce a patient's risk.

Such a technique must be able to precisely visualize the meniscus, as well as measure the right atrial depth on every patient. The jugular venous ultrasound studies discussed thus far demonstrate that with minimal training, a simple bedside technique to visualize the jugular vein and identify the meniscus has high diagnostic accuracy and is possible in any patient regardless of body size or neck thickness. However, they all still rely on the same five-centimeter right atrial depth assumption which invariably fails.

While this hybrid technique is superior to visual inspection, it is still not precise enough to substitute for a right heart catheterization. To overcome this limitation, physicians in the department of ultrasound diagnostics at the Tangdu Hospital in Shaanxi, China used the built-in measuring capabilities of ultrasound to show that they could "locate the center of the [right atrium] precisely based on solid geometry" and approximate right atrial depth with a high degree of accuracy. It involved a cumbersome but clever technique involving multiple people, an ultrasound probe, a pencil, and a ruler. The results were then added to the distance from the sternum to the height of the meniscus to come up with an estimated right atrial pressure. When compared to a central venous catheter measurement, they were astoundingly accurate, only off by 0.2 centimeters on average.[184] "The precise measurement of [right atrial pressure]," they conclude "was realized by accurately locating the collapse point of the [internal jugular vein] and the center of the [right atrium] by ultrasound." Though still not practical for a routine physical exam, this method clearly shows how precise ultrasound can be for estimating right atrial pressures.

In a similar but simplified method pioneered by the author of this book, a two-minute, two-step bedside ultrasound technique may be just as effective. When compared to gold standard right heart catheterization data, using an easier to identify landmark that corresponds to the center of the right atrium (Figure 14) combined with the determination if the internal jugular vein is distended at the supraclavicular point, elevated right atrial pressures can be ruled out with 90% sensitivity and 96% negative predictive value, making the decision to use diuretics far more objective.[185] Though confirmatory studies are needed before such a simple method could become mainstream, it is extremely easy to perform and could completely replace the JVP guesswork at the bedside.

Why Measuring the JVP Matters

Since the circulatory system is all interconnected, the JVP, which estimates right atrial pressure, is often utilized as a surrogate for cardiac pressures elsewhere. If it is high, it is assumed to be high everywhere else. This is the essence of why such an insanely clever technique has remained the bedrock of our physical exam for nearly 100 years, and why accurate measurement of the JVP is so important. However, just as with the right atrial depth assumption, this proxy measurement is not as precise as we would hope.

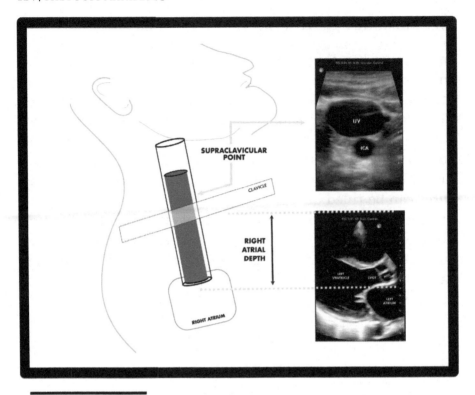

FIGURE 14

Simplified method by Istrail et al for estimating right atrial depth. The location where the non coronary cusp (NCC) of the aortic valve inserts on the posterior wall of the left ventricular outflow tract (LVOT) is used as surrogate for right atrium because it sits in the same coronal plane. It is also a very simple measurement to make with the patient supine. Then the internal jugular vein (IJV) is assessed for jugular venous distention (JVD). If JVD is present, it suggests the right atrial pressure is higher than the right atrial depth.

CHAPTER 15: PULMONARY CAPILLARY WEDGE PRESSURE & THE LVEDP

"The circulation should be kept as tranquil as possible by a strictly quiet life, and a moderate, unstimulating diet. The food, however, should be nutritious, comprising slightly under-dressed animal food, principally mutton and beef, twice a day, at breakfast and dinner, in order to keep the muscular system in general, and that of the heart in particular, in good tone."

DR. JAMES HOPE ON TREATING CONGESTIVE HEART FAILURE, 1839

In 1966, Dr. J Ward Kennedy, a pioneer in cardiovascular research at the University of Washington published *The Normal Left Ventricle in Man*,[186] measuring the volume and mass of normal hearts in 22 men and women. He and his co-authors measured the heart in ***diastole***, when it is relaxing and filling with blood, and compared it to ***systole*** when the blood is ejected.

They showed that the ***stroke volume***, or volume of blood ejected with each beat, can be calculated by taking the difference between the volume of blood in the left ventricle at its fullest, called **end-diastolic volume**, and subtracting the volume at the end of systole when it is least full.

End diastolic volume - stroke volume = end systolic volume

They called this stroke volume to end-diastolic volume ratio the **ejection fraction** that demonstrated "a narrow range of variation with a mean of 0.67." This was one of the first studies to determine that the left ventricle of a normal heart pumps about 65% of the blood with each beat. Such a heart endowed with a normal ejection fraction facilitates a homeostatic hum of healthy organs and dry lungs. Yet if the ejection fraction is reduced by any reason, fluid can accumulate upstream like a ten-car pile-up on the highway and wreak havoc in its wake. Whether from a myocardial infarction, uncontrolled hypertension, or less commonly a viral infection, injury to the left ventricle can cause irreversible damage and a **reduced ejection fraction**. If it is weakened by 50% for example, then the heart would eject 50% less blood and therefore the new ejection fraction would drop to about half of normal, or 30%. This can increase the end-diastolic volume, since less blood is ejected with each beat, resulting in an increased pressure in the left ventricle. This is called the **left ventricular end-diastolic pressure**, or **LVEDP** for short, and it is the gold standard measurement to determine a patient's left-sided heart pressure and overall "fluid status."

The Proxy of the Surrogate of the Estimate

The LVEDP can be measured directly through a left heart catheterization, in which a catheter is inserted through an artery and advanced retrogradely into the left side of the heart. However, the LVEDP is more often estimated through a right heart catheterization, with the **wedge pressure** as its proxy. This highlights an important point in our physical examination: the jugular venous pressure is a surrogate for right atrial pressure, which is then a surrogate for the wedge pressure, which itself is a proxy for LVEDP. Down each rung of this hemodynamic ladder, the accuracy tends to diminish.

The concordance of right atrial pressure to wedge pressure is about 75%,[187–189] and may be closer to 66% in patients with high right-sided pressures.[190] Likewise, the wedge pressure can often be discordant with the LVEDP. Such disparities are particularly important in a condition like **pulmonary hypertension**, where the diagnosis and treatment change considerably based on the patient's left ventricular pressures.

If a patient undergoes a right heart catheterization and is found to have elevated pressures in the pulmonary artery but normal pressures everywhere else (inferred from the **wedge pressure**), they may be diagnosed with **pulmonary arterial hypertension (PAH)**. This is a disorder located exclusively in the pulmonary arteries and requires a unique set of therapies, many of which were miraculously developed by the founder of Sirius Satellite Radio after her 10-year-old daughter was diagnosed with PAH, a terminal diagnosis at the time.[4]

Since the wedge pressure is a robust estimate of left-sided pressures, a right heart catheterization is usually sufficient to make such a diagnosis. However, when researchers looked at patients with pulmonary arterial hypertension diagnosed with a right heart catheterization alone, they found that more than half of them would no longer meet the diagnostic criteria if the gold-standard LVEDP was used instead.[192] This discordance has been confirmed in other studies as well,[193–196] suggesting that in an ideal scenario, the LVEDP should be measured or estimated directly.

Estimating Wedge Pressure and LVEDP with Ultrasound

As discussed previously, in patients with a reduced ejection fraction the heart is unable to sufficiently pump the blood it receives and excess pressure builds up, increasing the LVEDP. This in turn causes a backlog of fluid that can leak into the lungs and cause pulmonary edema, which can be detected with lung rockets in multiple rib spaces. This rise in pressure and backflow increases the number of B-lines and lung rockets, theoretically in proportion to the LVEDP. Various studies have been undertaken to qualitatively estimate the wedge pressure or LVEDP indirectly and noninvasively with ultrasound, using Dr. Lichtenstein's A-lines and B-lines from Part I.

For example, the presence of a normal ejection fraction combined with A-lines was 100% sensitive for a normal wedge pressure in one study.[197] Similarly in another study, the wedge pressure was never high in patients with no lung rockets present either at rest[57] or with exercise.[198] Dr. Lichtenstein tested this B-line to wedge pressure correlation as well, and found that for wedge pressure under 18 mmHg, A-line pattern was 93% specific. However, it was only 50% sensitive, and B-lines were seen with both high and low wedge pressures.[199] A huge limitation to such studies though, is the fact that the wedge pressure can be discordant with LVEDP up to 50% of the time, and therefore a more accurate estimate of a patient's volume status would be achieved by comparing lung ultrasound findings to LVEDP directly.

Physicians in France completed such a study, performing a lung ultrasound on 81 patients with shortness of breath prior to a left heart catheterization and formal echocardiogram.[200] Surprisingly, they found that none of the standard parameters measured with a formal echocardiogram correlated well with elevated LVEDP. In contrast, they discovered that in patients with high LVEDP over 20mmHg, the median B-line count was 17.0, while in those with normal LVEDP it was only 1.0. This B-line count was the variable "most strongly correlated with invasively measured LVEDP, and significantly increased both diagnostic accuracy and reclassification for elevated LVEDP." Zero patients with normal LVEDP had two or more lung rockets, while eight or more total B-lines were 90% specific and 78% sensitive for elevated LVEDP. Overall, in combination with the patient's cardiac history and presenting symptoms, eight or more B-lines had an *area under the curve* of 93.6%, corresponding to an outstanding ability to discriminate between patients with low and high LVEDP,[201] demonstrating the important capacity of B-lines to predict high left-sided heart pressures.

Managing Heart Failure Patients in the *POCUS Era*

In the *POCUS Era*, the diagnosis and management of congestive heart failure take on a more objective ideal. With the lessons already discussed, the traditional signs we use in the *Before POCUS era* can be improved upon to guide therapies with more precision. From Chapter 14, we know that POCUS offers a more accurate method for estimating the jugular venous pressure and corresponding right atrial pressure. The meniscus can be viewed in every patient regardless of body size, and using a basic sonographic exam can essentially rule out elevated pressures.[185] From the lessons of Dr. Lichtenstein in Part I, we know with 97% sensitivity and specificity[66] that if lung rockets and lung sliding are present in multiple rib spaces in both lungs, the patient has pulmonary edema and would likely benefit from diuretic therapy. We also know that eight or more B-lines in a patient with basic clinical characteristics of heart failure is more predictive of an elevated LVEDP than any other non-invasive echo technique we have. In congestive heart failure patients, we know that the number of B-lines correlates well with BNP levels, as well as the New York Heart Association's symptom classifications and that with adequate diuresis, B-line count reduces as symptoms improve.[202] In patients with shortness of breath and suspected heart failure, we know that with just basic cardiac POCUS, non-cardiologists can accurately diagnose a reduced ejection fraction and expedite care accordingly.

Overall, these techniques offer objective, noninvasive hemodynamic assessment of our heart failure patients, practices that lead to improved real-world outcomes. For example, in one study 123 heart failure patients were randomized to receive diuretic therapy guided by either standard physical examination or B-line count with lung ultrasound. Subjects who had their therapy guided by lung ultrasound overall received more diuretics, had less urgent care visits for heart failure symptoms, and had improved distance achieved in the 6-minute walk test.[203] Very similar results were seen in a 2020 randomized trial of 126 heart failure patients where those subjects in the lung ultrasound-guided treatment arm had a 45% reduction in urgent care visits for heart failure related causes compared to the physical-exam-only group.[204]

Also in 2020, Italian physicians studied 244 patients with heart failure in a multi-center trial that also randomized patients to a traditional physical exam guided therapy, or one with a physical exam and lung ultrasound. At 90-day follow-up, the patients who had lung-ultrasound-guided care had improvement in their BNP biomarker and quality of life questionnaire. More importantly, only 12 patients in the ultrasound group were hospitalized compared to 25 in the physical exam only group, a relative risk reduction of 56% with lung ultrasound. This led them to conclude that lung POCUS "improved the management of patients with chronic [heart failure]," and that lung ultrasound's accuracy "in detecting subclinical [pulmonary congestion] provides the possibility to tackle an early decompensation phase," reducing admissions for acute heart failure exacerbations, heart failure biomarkers and improving quality of life at 90-day follow up.[205]

Not only does cardiopulmonary POCUS improve our accuracy and objectivity, it results in measurable benefits for our real-life patients. Such results simply cannot be achieved by visual inspection of the neck veins, listening for pulmonary edema with accuracy approximating a coin-flip, or inferring the ejection fraction from a third heart sound. In the *POCUS Era*, we no longer need to pontificate on a patient's 'volume status' or degree of pulmonary edema. We can just look inside and know for sure. Could this be the beginning of the end of our eternal volume exam frustrations?

CHAPTER 16: PERICARDITIS, PERICARDIAL EFFUSIONS & TAMPONADE

"If the amount of effusion be sufficient to enfeeble the heart by compression, it is highly important to effect the removal of the liquid as speedily as possible. For this end, the precordia may be painted daily with the tincture of iodine, or small blisters may be applied, removing them as soon as vesication begins, and allowing the blistered surface to dry rapidly."

DR. AUSTIN FLINT ON THE TREATMENT OF PERICARDIAL
EFFUSIONS, 1881

Just as the lungs are encased in a bony thorax, the heart is enclosed in the *pericardium*, a fibrinous sack comprised of a durable connective tissue exterior surrounding an inner lining lubricated with 10-50 milliliters of pericardial fluid.[206] This pericardium offers a safe haven for the heart, a private enclosure walled off from pulmonary infection where it is free to complete its century of work. Yet this cardiac sanctuary can quickly become a place of peril if more than 50 milliliters of fluid rapidly accumulates inside. *Pericarditis* or inflammation of the pericardium is one condition that can result in this excess fluid accumulation. The heart's function can be compromised, as Dr. James Hope explained, "by the compression exercised by the fluid ... first, because the effusion is sudden, and organs do not so easily accommodate themselves to sudden, as to gradual compression." In addition, the pericardium is "deprived of its distensibility by inflammation," and is unable to expand to accept this invasive fluid. "Hence the heart, unable to transmit - perhaps even to receive, the blood, flutters, intermits, beats feebly, irregularly, and unequally...If this state be not expeditiously relieved by remedies, the patient dies in the space of a few days or even hours."[18] This external compression of the chambers of the heart that Hope described results in what we now know as *cardiac tamponade.*

These pericardial effusions and the pericarditis that often accompany them commonly develop covertly, or in the presence of nonspecific symptoms like chest discomfort, fevers, or shortness of breath, making it a challenging diagnosis to make. "There is no inflammatory affection of which the diagnosis has been considered more difficult than pericarditis," described Hope. "Laennec states that he has often ... discovered the disease in a severe form, when nothing had afforded a suspicion of its existence; and, on the other hand, that he has frequently witnessed all its signs, without finding a vestige of the malady."

Dr. Jean Nicolas Corvisart who first popularized the percussion techniques felt it could be detected with "heat in the region of the heart; great difficulty of respiration; greater colour of the left cheek than the right," though Laennec did not appreciate these findings. Humbled by the difficult diagnosis, Laennec believed pericarditis is "as frequently mistaken as recognised," and that "the stethoscope scarcely furnishes us with any more certain signs of this disease."[1]

Yet Dr. Hope did note a murmur with his stethoscope that may be heard at the start of pericarditis before significant fluid has accumulated, which has since been termed a *pericardial friction rub*. It "is almost always double, accompanying the two sounds of the heart, in correspondence with the movements of the organ backwards and forwards within the pericardium." He described the murmur as having a "rough character, sometimes like the rasping of wood, or the grating of a nutmeg," and that rarely it resembles "the creaking of a new shoe-sole."

Hope's diagnostic description of pericardial effusions and tamponade were impressively accurate, yet his recommended treatments were comically characteristic of the time. When treating pericarditis, he noted that "blood should ... be drawn freely and by a large incision ... so as to bring [the patient] to the verge of syncope. From five and twenty to forty leeches, according to the strength should be applied to the precordial region ... The intestinal canal, if at all confined, should immediately be evacuated by a purgative enema." Both of these 'treatments,' as we now know, would have the opposite effect and expedite death.

Cardiac Tamponade & Beck's Triad

Approximately 100 years later, even as the understanding of pericardial effusions and possible therapies were advancing, Dr. Claude Beck, a pioneering American cardiac surgeon from the early 20th century, still felt diseases of the pericardium were "generally difficult problems in diagnosis." He devised a 'cardiac compression triad' (later known as *Beck's triad*) to help doctors with this clinical conundrum. They consisted of "(1) falling blood pressure, (2) rising venous pressure and (3) a small quiet heart," and he felt that "all other clinical manifestations of acute compression are secondary to this triad."[207] He explained that when the heart is being externally compressed, "the great venous gateway to the heart ... is partially or completely collapsed. The ventricles are also smaller than normal. The heart, being partially collapsed, is able to make only a feeble excursion." Even a small effusion could be dangerous, he explained, noting that "if the compression is due to intrapericardial hemorrhage and develops acutely ... as little as 200 cc. of blood may be fatal."

To this day, Dr. Beck's triad is taught to medical trainees learning how to detect cardiac tamponade. However, what exactly does 'a small quiet heart' mean? Is low blood pressure seen in all cases or few? And how does Dr. Beck's triad compare to Gunther's rusty lobster catcher?

Tamponade, a "clinical diagnosis"

In the *Before POCUS era*, since there is no simple way to look at the heart and pericardium, it is commonly taught that pericardial tamponade is a "clinical diagnosis," meaning that it is primarily diagnosed based on the signs and symptoms that can be appreciated at the bedside with a stethoscope. This concept has been bludgeoned into the brains of countless trainees who suggest ordering an echocardiogram instead, based on the assumption that the clinical exam findings are sensitive and specific enough to make the diagnosis on their own. Yet the most common presenting symptoms are shortness of breath and chest pain,[208] neither of which is specific enough to pinpoint the cause. Likewise, the most commonly cited signs of pericardial tamponade - hypotension, tachycardia, diminished heart sounds, elevated jugular venous pressure, and pulsus paradoxus - may not be sensitive or specific enough either.

Low blood pressure

Beck's triad states that patients with tamponade experience low blood pressure. While this is certainly true in the late stages of tamponade, the hemodynamics in less acute cases are not so clear-cut. Contrary to Beck's triad, University of Cincinnati Medical Center physicians reported on 56 patients with tamponade, noting they "were not in a shock-like state: 64% had an average systolic arterial blood pressure greater than 100mmHg."[209] These findings are similar to data from a large Canadian hospital in patients with tamponade requiring drainage, where they found low blood pressure only 10% of the time.[208] This was also true at a hospital in Birmingham, England where only 25% of tamponade patients were hypotensive,[210] as well as in a Harvard Medical School study where the mean systolic blood pressure was 123 mmHg and only 14% were hypotensive.[211] In fact, multiple studies have demonstrated that patients can even present with *elevated* blood pressure and still have cardiac tamponade.[212–214]

Tachycardia

Tachycardia is certainly a concerning finding in a patient with tamponade, suggesting the heart is struggling to eject sufficient amounts of blood to the body. However, it is very common in hospitalized patients and therefore has very low specificity, and may be blunted by the high percentage of patients that are on heart rate lowering medications such as beta-blockers. Nevertheless, it is present between 68%[215] and 77%[216] of patients with known tamponade.

Rising Venous Pressure

As the pressure in the pericardial sac rises, the venous drainage is prevented from entering the heart, causing it to back up and engorge the veins. Elevated jugular venous pressure (JVP) was present in 50%[215] to 76%[216] of patients, a number that is almost certainly an underestimation due to our poor ability to detect JVP visually, as discussed previously. Of course, elevated JVP is not specific to cardiac tamponade either, often being present in congestive heart failure, for example.

Diminished Heart Sounds

This finding is particularly difficult to assess objectively and is a clear relic of the *Before POCUS Era*. Diminished compared to what? The volume of the heart sounds are confounded by multiple factors including body size and ambient noise present. In studies that did attempt to determine if the heart sounds were diminished, it was only 28% sensitive for tamponade.[216]

Pulsus Paradoxus

In patients without a pericardial effusion compressing their heart, there is a normal physiologic decrease in systolic blood pressure of 10 mmHg or less during inspiration. This drop is amplified during cardiac compression, and a decrease of more than 10 mmHg is called *pulsus paradoxus*, a clever finding that can be used to detect the presence of tamponade. According to an early study of 65 patients, pulsus paradoxus can detect tamponade with 98% sensitivity,[217] while a review article and meta-analysis of eight studies from 2007 in the *Journal of the American Medical Association* pegged it at 82%.[216] In a study of 46 patients over a 10 year period at a hospital in the UK the sensitivity and specificity of pulsus paradoxus was 80% and 100% respectively,[210] while in an earlier study from the 1980s using right heart catheterization pressures as the gold standard, the sensitivity and specificity was only 79% and 40% respectively.[218] While pulsus paradoxus can be very useful in diagnosing cardiac tamponade, it can also be seen in other conditions like right ventricular infarction, hypovolemia, constrictive pericarditis, restrictive cardiomyopathy, pneumothorax, COPD, bilateral pleural effusions, asthma, and pulmonary embolism.[219,220]

Diagnosing Tamponade in the POCUS Era

A major limitation to Beck's triad is that its criteria are also seen in many other cardiac or pulmonary conditions besides tamponade. A patient with mild hypotension and tachycardia who has pneumonia is less urgent than one with those same vital signs that has a large pericardial effusion. In the *POCUS Era*, however, an ultrasound can be placed on that patient's chest and the existence of a pericardial effusion can be known with certainty in a matter of seconds. The absence of such fluid by definition excludes tamponade,[221] while the presence of a pericardial effusion makes the clinical findings of Beck's Triad or pulsus paradoxus far more useful.

If there is fluid present, then its hindrance upon the heart must be assessed. If the pressures against the heart are sufficiently high, then as Dr. Beck explained, the veins will be unable to drain into the right atrium and the pressure in the veins emptying into the heart will rise. This can be detected in the internal jugular vein (as we have seen in congestive heart failure), as well as with a POCUS exam of the *inferior vena cava* (IVC), that returns blood from the lower portion of the body back into the right heart. If there is external compression of the right atrium from pericardial fluid, the IVC will be dilated. If the pressure is sufficiently high in the IVC, just as in the jugular veins, its normal collapsibility with each breath will be blunted. This is called *IVC plethora*, and like Gunther's upgraded lobster catcher, it picks up 97% of tamponade cases,[222] therefore, if it is not present, tamponade can essentially be ruled out. It is often the first echocardiographic sign to appear and the last to resolve after pericardial drainage and has the highest predictive accuracy of cardiac tamponade when compared to other echocardiographic signs.[223] It is not specific though, since any condition that increases cardiac pressures can cause IVC plethora.[221]

Right-Sided Collapse

As the effusion accumulates, the pressure in the pericardium increases. When this pressure exceeds the internal cardiac chamber pressures, the heart's walls will begin to collapse. This occurs in escalating order of each chamber's internal pressure. Since the right atrium and ventricle have the thinnest walls with the lowest internal pressures, the earliest signs of tamponade will be seen in these right heart chambers.

The location and time with the lowest pressure in the heart is the *right atrium during ventricular systole*, and therefore the first place where compression would be evident. Instead of maintaining its dome-like shape during systole (when the tricuspid valve is closed), its wall can invert from the external pressure. The longer it remains inappropriately inverted when it is supposed to be filling with blood during systole, the more likely tamponade is to be present. If it is more than ⅓ of systole it is 94% sensitive and 100% specific for tamponade,[221] however, determining this at the bedside can be difficult especially in the setting of tachycardia.

The next lowest pressure location is the *right ventricle during diastole* (when the tricuspid valve is open). As the right ventricle is filling, it should be fully expanded to accept its dollop of blood to send to the lungs. Therefore, if the right ventricular wall during this time is compressed inward, it is abnormal. Since the pressure required to collapse the right ventricle during systole is slightly higher than the atrium, the sensitivity is somewhat less (60 to 90%) though it is more specific (85 to 100%) as compared to *brief* right atrial collapse.[221]

These POCUS signs of tamponade can be simplified into three statements:

1. Inferior vena cava plethora without regular respiratory variation
2. Right atrial collapse when the tricuspid valve is closed
3. Right ventricle collapse when the tricuspid valve is open

Yet even without determining diastolic or systolic collapse, just a general gestalt of how the right ventricular wall is contracting in the presence of pericardial fluid can provide clues that tamponade may be on the horizon. If the right ventricle appears to be flapping in the wind, here on referred to as the *air dancer sign* for its resemblance to the inflatable products outside car dealerships, then it is probably struggling to pump effectively. Also described as "a little man jumping on a trampoline,"[224] this is a sign of possible right ventricular distress that warrants a formal echocardiogram and a cardiology consult at the least.

Time is Life

The reason POCUS is so important in cases of pericardial effusions is that early recognition of tamponade results in earlier treatment and lives saved. In a large study comparing POCUS to traditional echocardiograms, the average time to diagnosis was 5.9 hours and the time to drainage was 28 hours in the POCUS group, while with traditional echocardiograms it was 45 hours and 49 hours respectively.[208] Similar results were seen at an emergency department in Israel, where POCUS-diagnosed tamponade had less fluid accumulation at the time of drainage, was drained in 11 hours as opposed to 70, and resulted in earlier discharge from the hospital.[225]

It is clear, therefore, that for accurate detection and timely treatment, tamponade is a clinical *and POCUS* diagnosis. Without knowing what is, or isn't, lurking in the pericardium, the common exam findings are not sensitive or specific enough. With the high stakes, time-sensitive decisions that tamponade requires, art and tradition should take a backseat to precision and certainty. Therefore, in the *POCUS Era*, a bedside cardiac ultrasound should be incorporated into every history and physical exam in a patient with suspected pericarditis, pericardial effusion, or tamponade. There is just no good reason not to.

PART III

CRITICISM & PRAISE

"When a distinguished but elderly scientist states that something is possible, he is almost certainly right. When he states that something is impossible, he is very probably wrong."

"Every revolutionary idea seems to evoke three stages of reaction. They may be summed up by the phrases: (1) It's completely impossible. (2) It's possible, but it's not worth doing. (3) I said it was a good idea all along."

ARTHUR C. CLARKE

1917 - 2008

CHAPTER 17: POCUS IN THE HORSELESS AGE

"Talking of horseless carriage suggests to my mind that the horse is doomed. The bicycle, which, 10 years ago, was a curiosity, is now a necessity. It is found everywhere. Ten years from now you will be able to buy a horseless vehicle for what you would pay today for a wagon and a pair of horses. The money spent in the keep of the horses will be saved and the danger to life will be much reduced. It is only a question of a short time when the carriages and trucks of every large city will be run by motors. The expense of keeping and feeding horses in a great city like New York is very heavy, and all this will be done away with. You must remember that every invention of this kind which is made adds to the general wealth by introducing a new system of greater economy of force. A great invention which facilitates commerce, enriches a country just as much as the discovery of vast hoards of gold."

THOMAS EDISON, 1895

At the end of the 19th century, the horse and buggy was the standard method of transportation in the United States. Bicycles were popular as well, and the founder of Winton Bicycle Co, Alexander Winton, had visions of better transportation. He pondered the possibility of a self-propelling upgrade to his bikes that would use gasoline,226 envisioning "something a rider wouldn't have to push and keep pushing if he was trying to get someplace." The biggest obstacle to widespread adoption of such an automobile, he thought, was "the lack of public interest. To advocate replacing the horse, which had served man through centuries, marked one as an imbecile." Even someone like him, with a successful bicycle business would be pointed out as "the fool who is fiddling with a buggy that will run without being hitched to a horse." His banker told him "you're crazy if you think this fool contraption you've been wasting your time on will ever displace the horse." Fortunately for the future of humanity, Winton did not cede to his shortsighted critics and in 1897 he founded the Winton Motor Carriage Company, one of the first American companies to manufacture a motor car.

The prospects of a new type of vehicle powered by motor rather than horse brought fear and fear-mongering among government officials and engineers at the time, arguments analogous to those against POCUS today. A London engineering magazine spoke of "slaughtered pedestrians and shattered vehicles" that would occur if cars were allowed on the roads.[227] They feared the cars would be driven by amateurs rather than people with extra "mechanical training." The inference from these statements, wrote the authors of a pro-motorized-vehicle newsletter called *The Horseless Age*, is that "only persons of "mechanical training" know the laws of the road, and only they are to be entrusted with the guidance of a motor vehicle. But how is it with horse vehicles? Are all careful drivers persons of "mechanical training?" ... A man must become familiar with the management of any machine in order to handle it successfully on the road, but this applies as well to a horse as to a motor."

Similar dissension echoed from the pages of the prestigious medical journal *Chest* twelve decades later in a back-and-forth discussion regarding the appropriate use of POCUS. Doctors from Denmark asserted that POCUS should not be used in place of a stethoscope.[228] Many of the findings on lung ultrasound, they explained, "may be caused by a range of pathologies ... As such, apart from being able to perform POCUS, the clinician must be able to assess and integrate the sonographic data with any other available clinical information to come to a working diagnosis and treatment plan. This leaves POCUS in the breathless patient vulnerable to the skill of the operator in acquiring and interpreting ultrasound images, as well as to their clinical judgment and ability to use this additional information to actually inform the diagnosis and not simply succumb to confirmation bias." This is true of course, but no different than with using a stethoscope. Auscultation findings are subject to the skill of the operator and confirmation bias as well.

"We believe that some truths are self-evident," wrote Drs. Koenig and Tsegaye in a rebuttal.[229] "POCUS should be performed by the clinical provider and that provider must have training to competency. We believe all physicians who take care of patients who are acutely short of breath should have these skills. No one would allow a physician who doesn't know how to use a stethoscope to take care of patients. But how do we know that those clinicians know what they are hearing? ... We believe that POCUS is an extension of the physical examination, that the device is more sensitive and specific than the stethoscope and therefore all should know how to use it."

Those arguing for maintaining the stethoscope status quo go on to say that for POCUS to be incorporated into routine practice, it would require "evidence of a positive impact on clinical care or improvement of hard outcomes like reduction in patient morbidity and mortality, or use of health-care resources." Such data is absent with POCUS, they argue, and therefore "cannot be regarded yet as a standard of care."

An English group of physicians responded, arguing that we should not conflate "the concept of an intervention, which is designed to improve patient outcomes, with a diagnostic test, which is expected to improve diagnostic accuracy. POCUS is the latter: a diagnostic test that has demonstrated improved accuracy vs both chest radiograph and auscultation in a number of situations ... We do not advocate chest CT scan in complex cases because it improves outcomes; we advocate it because it improves diagnostic accuracy. This is the standard that needs to be met, and the standard that POCUS arguably already exceeds."[230]

Inherent in these arguments against POCUS is the assumption that our current standard of care - the stethoscope - already provides robust diagnostic accuracy and improves morbidity and mortality, an argument not supported in the medical literature. There is no question that adequate training needs to be provided to clinicians before they are able to use POCUS independently. Or as Koenig and Tesgaye phrased it: "A fool is still a fool, with ultrasound or without." A clinician "must know how to integrate the ultrasound findings into the clinical picture; otherwise it is just another radiologic study where "clinical correlation" will be advised."

This ongoing debate has played out in the media as well. In 2016, Dr. Sanjiv Kaul, the head of the division of cardiovascular medicine at the Oregon Health and Science University, thought it was "time to discard the inaccurate, albeit iconic, stethoscope and join the rest of mankind in the technology revolution," he explained in a Washington Post article, arguing instead that we should focus on the abilities of handheld ultrasound. "We are not at the place, and probably won't be for a very long time," countered Dr. W. Reid Thompson, an associate professor of pediatrics at Johns Hopkins University School of Medicine, "where listening to the body's sounds is replaced by imaging."[231] This may have been true at the time, though just 20 months later the FDA would approve the first handheld full-body, smartphone-connected ultrasound device, ushering in the the POCUS Era that Dr. Kaul presciently described.[232]

Modern Day POCUS and its Criticisms

This civil discourse is essential to deciding if such a new technology should be incorporated into our daily medical practice. Equally important though in our quest to improve patient care, should be a willingness to embrace such technologies in the face of overwhelming evidence. As discussed throughout this book, whether it be Alexander Winton and his horseless buggy, Laennec with his stethoscope, Dr. Hope with more precise cardiac auscultation, Lichtenstein and lung ultrasound, or Feigenbaum and echo, the initial reception was more consistent with dismissive pushback and ridicule rather than healthy skepticism and open-mindedness. This resistance to change may be part of our human condition, a knee-jerk response from practitioners of the status quo that is still present today. It manifests as some variation of the idea that POCUS, or other such diagnostic novelties, are a distraction pursued by the technology-obsessed generation of clinicians whose clinical abilities are "not like they used to be." Or, as an internal medicine physician described it in an article acerbically titled *Hyposkilia: Deficiency of Clinical Skills:*[233]

> *"While modern medical technology has greatly enhanced our ability to diagnose and treat disease, it has also promoted laziness—especially mental laziness—among many physicians. Habitual reliance on sophisticated medical gadgetry for diagnosis prevents physicians from using the most sophisticated, intricate machine they'll ever and always have—the brain."*

Such arguments are correct to some degree, as our over-reliance on excessive imaging has certainly dulled our physical exam skills. But ubiquitously absent from such condescension from the old medical guard is a turn of the microscope upon their own preconceived notions. An objective rather than a nostalgic look at the data supporting the medical traditions they hold so dearly. Or, as biologist Thomas Henry Huxley put it in a speech at the founding of Johns Hopkins University in 1876: "Sit down before a fact as a little child, be prepared to give up every preconceived notion, follow humbly wherever and to whatever abysses nature leads, or you shall learn nothing."[234] Unfortunately, this objective inquiry into the data supporting many examination techniques is often beat down as blasphemy since the stethoscope-based physical exam is viewed by some as a medical ritual that dare not be questioned.

As dangerous as this hypothetical trainee that "doesn't use their brain" may be, our overreliance on outdated, imprecise measures combined with overconfidence in our own clinical skills can be equally as damaging to a patient's health. As cardiologist and POCUS pioneer Dr. Roelandt put it: "we should recognize that most of us never were able to match the talents and skills of the master teachers, and that our examination skills gradually decline with time and age."[235] He felt that the increased reliance of the younger generation on bedside ultrasound in place of our 200-year-old stethoscopic exams should be encouraged, not suppressed:

> "Is it not logical that they want to obtain as much objective information as possible when they first see the patients? Small hand carried ultrasound imaging devices offer the potential to achieve this desire. These devices can be used anywhere just like a conventional stethoscope. They should not replace the physical examination but significantly increase its yield and accuracy at first contact with the patient by extending our physical sense of seeing and recognising (major) cardiac abnormalities."

As recently as 2021, the *Journal of the American Medical Association* published an editorial on POCUS,[236] reiterating many of the same criticisms voiced by clinicians in *Chest* described earlier. "There is no doubt that POCUS use is viscerally satisfying and appeals to the clinician taking care of patients," the authors wrote, however, "many unanswered questions remain with regard to its use." They argued the clinical benefit is challenged by the fact that "these examinations are often performed without formal documentation, and images may not be easily accessed for quality assurance and retrospective analysis." While they are correct that POCUS may be used by clinicians that do not document their findings, this is a criticism of the clinician rather than the diagnostic modality itself. There is already significant literature and guidelines published on POCUS documentation, billing, and appropriate use.[237,238] And yes, ideally all images captured should be uploaded to the patient's chart, a practice many hospitals are rapidly adopting. Yet this criticism is also true of the stethoscope. There is no way to assess for quality assurance and retrospectively analyze a given patient's auscultation findings, the nuances of which are arguably harder to master than POCUS.

The authors go on to express concern over the lack of "meaningful clinical outcomes related to POCUS or even indirect clinical outcomes, such as time to treatment initiation, avoidance of transfer to a higher level of care, or length of stay." This of course ignores the fact that those certainly don't exist for the stethoscope, our current standard of care, either. It also mistakes POCUS for a medical intervention rather than a superior diagnostic tool, and fails to include studies that *have* shown improved clinical outcomes in heart failure management for example,[203–205] or time to pericardiocentesis in cardiac tamponade as discussed earlier.[208,225]

As witnessed by the dozens of negative comments on an editorial written about POCUS by the author of this book in 2020, other criticisms stem from the worry that introducing POCUS would diminish the physical exam and destroy the physician-patient relationship,[239] concerns that are largely unfounded. POCUS is a bedside diagnostic technique that allows the clinician to peer into the body and visually inspect the internal organs during their physical exam. It is a modern-day tool with better sensitivity and specificity than the stethoscope or the chest X-ray, and it improves - not harms - the relationship with the patient. In a Danish study of over 600 patients' perception of incorporating POCUS into their care, 45% reported it improved the doctor-patient relationship and more than half felt they were taken more seriously. 92% felt they were more thoroughly examined and 95% reported that POCUS improved their overall level of care.[240]

This is not to say that the stethoscope does not still provide value in certain situations. Those excited about POCUS - including yours truly - should also acknowledge the benefits a stethoscope may still have over ultrasound. While the price of a personal ultrasound device has reduced considerably, a stethoscope is still far cheaper and doesn't need to be charged, connected to a phone, or plugged into a power outlet. It does have good specificity for ruling in a limited set of diseases such as a large pneumothorax, isolated aortic stenosis, isolated mitral regurgitation, or to detect wheezing. It also can be a lot easier to use in small babies or to simply detect the presence of breath sounds after intubation, and already has the training component built into the medical education. However, if we can now peer inside the body and view the inner workings of our internal organs that a stethoscope can merely infer, is it not a useful tool that we should utilize?

CHAPTER 18: POCUS
USE TODAY

"Half of what you'll learn in medical school will be shown to be either dead wrong or out of date within five years of your graduation; the trouble is that nobody can tell you which half."

DR. DAVE SACKET, PIONEER OF EVIDENCE-BASED MEDICINE

It is difficult to fully grasp the potential POCUS can offer to the clinician-patient relationship without experiencing it firsthand. While focused ultrasound exams have been accepted in emergency medicine for many years, it has yet to reach a critical mass in other specialties like internal medicine. Whether it is general internal medicine, nephrology, or critical-care, POCUS offers a large spectrum of opportunities to improve diagnostic accuracy, prevent unnecessary tests and procedures, and dramatically change a patient's clinical experience.

For Dr. Renee Dversdal, a hospitalist physician and Chief Medical Officer of Vave Health, the process of incorporating POCUS into her practice was a gradual one (Figure 15). She saw the potential POCUS had and was learning how to use it. Then one night shift during her first year as an attending, she "had the true 'aha' moment and never looked back!" A patient was transferred from a rural hospital with the diagnosis of pneumonia, yet was not improving with antibiotics and IV fluids. Dr. Dversdal examined the patient and then ultrasounded their heart. When she cycled through different views of the heart, she found evidence of severe right heart strain concerning instead for a ***pulmonary embolism***. "I ran down to the ED and showed them the clips, as I still wasn't super confident." They agreed and the patient was sent for a CT scan which confirmed a large pulmonary embolus, not pneumonia.[241]

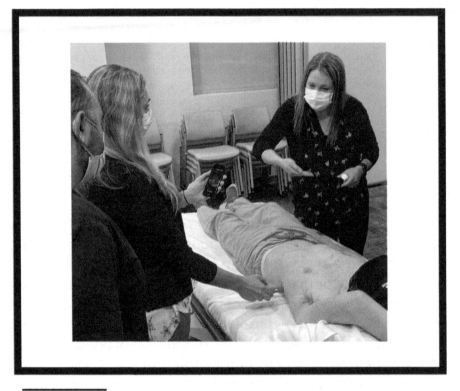

FIGURE 15   Hospitalist and CMO of Vave Health Dr. Renee Dversdal teaching lung ultrasound with wireless ultrasound probes. Masked due to the COVID-19 pandemic.

With permission from Dr. Dversdal

These U-turns in a patient's clinical trajectory after a bedside ultrasound exam are such a common experience among POCUS-wielding clinicians that they even have a name. Dr. Nilam Soni (Figure 16), a pioneer in the field of internal medicine POCUS and co-author of the seminal point-of-care ultrasound text-book,[32] calls it the "POCUS Kiss," or "PO-kiss" for short. Out of the hundreds of *PO-kisses* Soni has had in his career, one that stands out was a patient transferred to his hospital with multiple lesions in his lung and the diagnosis of "metastatic cancer likely needing hospice." Upon Dr. Soni's physical exam, he noted the patient's right thigh to be more swollen than the left. He placed the ultrasound probe on the patient's leg and immediately saw a large blood clot brewing in the common femoral vein. As it turned out, the patient had knee surgery one month prior, and the lung lesions were actually **pulmonary emboli.** "So he went from 'you have metastatic cancer and you're not going to live much longer,' to 'you have a large blood clot and portions broke off and got into your lung, and you will be better after a few months of anticoagulation.'"

To Soni, the utility of POCUS ultimately comes down to optimizing your time at the patient's bedside, and what information you can glean from your bedside evaluation. "We have the medical history that gets us in the ballpark. The history is very important, in many cases more important than the physical exam. And when you talk about examining the patients, we have the stethoscope, which is 200 years old. We have our hands and our reflex hammers which are not very sensitive. We are trying to make critical decisions about how to work up and manage a patient based on very rudimentary tools." So when Soni came across POCUS it changed everything.

His introduction to point-of-care ultrasound started as a third-year medical student on his trauma surgery rotation. At that time the FAST (Focused Assessment with Sonography in Trauma) exam had just come out, and the surgery residents were using ultrasound to quickly examine the abdomen and rule out signs of bleeding. Soni was impressed by this new protocol but wondered why they were not using ultrasound for non-trauma patients as well. In a patient with a suspected leg abscess he saw for example, "we cut into his thigh thinking he had an abscess, but he didn't have an abscess." Which, at the time he thought "Oh my God, that's terrible. We just cut into someone's leg and there's no abscess, nothing to drain. This poor old man is going to have to find somebody to help pack it. It's painful and he will have a scar on his leg. Why did we do that?"

No one he asked could give him a good answer "as to why we were not using [focused ultrasound] for other applications. And that's kind of where the curiosity really started." Soni looked into other point-of-care diagnostics, like rapid interpretation of electrolytes or procalcitonin blood tests, but with POCUS it "opened up a whole new arena of bedside diagnostics," and he was hooked.[242]

For hospitalist physicians in particular, Soni feels POCUS provides other invaluable functions: off-hours decision making and getting the attention of consultants. In 2006 he was working night shifts at the University of Chicago, and quickly realized that the daytime hospital during regular business hours is very different from the nighttime or weekend hospital. "There are 168 hours in a week. If the hospital is fully staffed and fully functional for let's say 50 hours per week, from 7 am till 5 pm every weekday, well that's still less than a third of the time that the hospital is fully staffed." The remaining time, he explained, has limited technicians or sonographers, and various specialists are only available by phone. Therefore, "this is where POCUS really comes in. It's not the cure-all, but it definitely helps bridge some of these gaps. For making decisions during the majority of time considered to be off-hours, it's a huge resource. It changes your decision-making and quickly narrows your differential diagnosis." Most importantly, noted Soni, "it gets the attention of consultants when needed."

In the case of pericardial effusions and tamponade, for example, "if you call the cardiologist on-call in the middle of the night and say 'Hey, you know I hear dull heart sounds, the blood pressure is kind of low, I think he might have tamponade,' they aren't going to pay attention to you," Soni said. "But if you send them an image of a large pericardial effusion in a patient who is hypotensive, that's all you've got to say. It will get their attention. An image says 1,000 words, as trite as that is. It's really powerful for what we are doing." Likewise, if you call the pulmonologist and say "this guy is short of breath. He's got some dullness to percussion, I think he has a large pleural effusion," Soni explains, "no one is going to respond with any urgency. But if you show them a picture of a large pleural effusion that needs drainage they'll say: Oh yeah, let's get him scheduled for a thoracentesis. So for any general internists, POCUS is really a great way to mobilize resources."

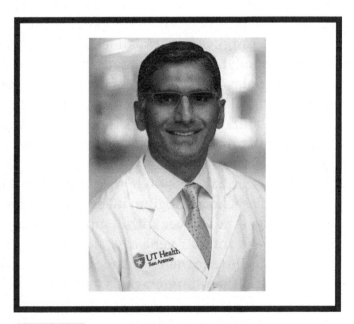

FIGURE 16 Dr. Nilam Soni, a pioneer in internal medicine POCUS and author of *Point-of-care Ultrasound*, the seminal POCUS textbook. He is now the leader of point-of-care ultrasound training at UT San Antonio and the VA health care system.

For specialists in internal medicine, POCUS provides value in other ways. Dr. Abhilash Koratala, a Nephrologist and assistant professor of Medicine at the Medical College of Wisconsin, uses POCUS because it allows for more precise and timely examination of his patients with kidney disease. He was a nephrology fellow at the University of Florida when he came across POCUS for the first time. He was seeing a consult in the emergency department and asked for an ultrasound "to exclude urinary obstruction; however, I was surprised to learn that the emergency physician had already performed it. Until then, I was not familiar with non-radiologist physicians performing ultrasound at the patient's bedside for anything other than procedural guidance. That incident piqued my interest in bedside ultrasonography."[243]

Dr. Koratala began learning kidney ultrasound by performing practice scans and comparing his findings with the radiology report. As his skills improved, he expanded to "POCUS-assisted comprehensive hemodynamic assessments," which he feels is crucial in his day-to-day nephrology practice. "POCUS helps me spend more meaningful time with patients, gather better histories, educate them about their condition," and is especially useful for providing instant answers to focused clinical questions. For example, if a dialysis patient under Dr. Koralata's care is suspected to have a pericardial effusion in the outpatient unit, "obtaining a consultative echocardiogram takes at least a few days," while Koralata can get the answer within minutes using POCUS. He also uses lung (and inferior vena cava) ultrasound to assess for B-lines and guide diuretic therapy, since they are much more sensitive and specific than lung crackles and lower extremity edema.

In terms of using a stethoscope, Dr. Koralata feels that for detecting wheezing, or a pericardial friction rub heard in some cases of pericarditis, "a stethoscope is clearly superior" since an ultrasound is unable to detect them. This sentiment was echoed by Dr. Dversdal, who still feels POCUS is "complementary rather than alternative to the stethoscope" for wheezes you can't ultrasound or regurgitant valves that are difficult to visualize.

In Koralata's nephrology practice, however, "it is rare to deal with patients who have symptomatic obstructive airway disease. Uremic pericarditis is considered an indication to initiate dialysis, but it is uncommon to see such patients these days with improved chronic kidney disease care. Moreover, while pericardial rub is specific for pericarditis, the sensitivity is relatively low. In these instances, POCUS can still help when coupled with good history taking and findings that are interpreted in the appropriate clinical context."

For acutely ill patients, POCUS plays a very powerful role as well. "I was drawn to acute medicine, and did a lot of critical care and community general medicine," explained Dr. Katie Wiskar, a POCUS fellowship-trained general internist from British Columbia, "and especially in these settings - the patient with undifferentiated hypotension or hypoxia for example - POCUS is just so game-changing. It seemed like a superpower to be able to instantly access that kind of information." After completing her POCUS fellowship and becoming an expert with an ultrasound probe, she has found less use for her stethoscope. "I will borrow one if I want to listen for a wheeze. However, I practice in an academic center with residents, so before I meet a patient, they've had a traditional screening physical exam with a stethoscope. I get to focus on where the money is - and, spoiler, it's the ultrasound." Ultimately, Dr. Wiskar uses POCUS because she feels it makes her a better clinician. "It gives me reliable, detailed information quickly and easily; and can be repeated serially in response to clinical change. The patients we care for these days are complex, and diagnoses are often not straightforward. POCUS is not the only answer - and it should always be incorporated and interpreted in conjunction with the rest of the clinical picture - but I really can't imagine practicing without it."[244]

In the intensive care unit, POCUS has a uniquely critical role in expediting diagnoses and tailoring treatments accordingly. Dr. Jonny Wilkinson, a consultant in intensive care and anesthesia in Northampton, United Kingdom, has had a similar experience as Dr. Wiskar. "Ultrasound is a no-brainer for me. It is like shining a torch into the patient and seeing things you could not see before."[245] In the noisy ICU environment where he works, the stethoscope is particularly difficult to use. He feels there is still a place for it to detect wheezing, but otherwise, Wilkinson relies entirely on POCUS. Being trained in anesthesia, he was already doing so many ultrasound-guided procedures, so "whole body POCUS seemed an obvious leap for me. I have never looked back! ... POCUS has hugely decreased my reliance on chest X-rays," only ordering them to confirm central line placement, and only ordering formal echocardiograms if he has a very specific clinical question his bedside POCUS cannot answer. "Ultrasound has become an indispensable cog in the machinery of my clinical examination subset. Inspection, palpation, percussion, and auscultation are forever complemented with insonation; almost to the degree of the death of percussion and auscultation." Wilkinson often wonders if we "will ever see just a triad of examinations appearing in our lifetimes: inspection, palpation, and insonation?"[246]

Like Wilkinson, Dr. Olusegun Olusanya, a London-based intensive care physician and Focused Ultrasound in Intensive Care Supervisor, uses his stethoscope very sparingly. "I don't think auscultation is completely dead. It's familiar, it has high specificity, it still detects wheeze, and it can be a useful screening tool prior to finalizing your diagnosis," but in Olusanya's practice, he uses POCUS almost exclusively. He first discovered point-of-care ultrasound when he was a first year physician. "I saw my cardiology registrar - a chief resident in American currency - learning how to echo. It was my 'Aha' moment of 'wow this stuff isn't just for radiologists!" The next year a cardiac physiologist showed him some basic echo techniques that he began using on his patients. "I picked up a high output heart failure, and I was hooked." Whether for procedural guidance or diagnostic imaging, he now uses POCUS for everything from focused echocardiograms or lung exams, to leg exams looking for deep vein thromboses, to even transcranial ultrasound to look at the cerebral blood vessels. "If you work with unstable patients, perform invasive procedures, and potentially have delays in getting imaging, POCUS is a no-brainer. Why would you continue guessing that there was pleural fluid based on reduced breath sounds and dullness to percussion when you can instantly know with nearly 100% certainty that there was one, how much fluid there was, and how easy it would be to drain with a simple device at the bedside?"

Integrating Ultrasound into Medical Education

On August 9, 2019, the new medical students at UC Irvine School of Medicine arrived for their white coat ceremony, ready to don their new attire in the annual tradition of medical education. "At UC Irvine, you guys graduate with special powers that most other medical students don't have," said Chair of Emergency Medicine and director of ultrasound in medical education, Dr. Chris Fox, from the stage. "The medical community will know that UCI graduates will be able to "not just do a history and physical exam," but "actually be able to look into the entire body from the eyeballs all the way down to the heel of the foot."[247] After a live demonstration of what a handheld ultrasound device attached to a smartphone is capable of, the dean of the medical school, Dr. Michael Stamos, took the stage for the keynote address. "We put a lot of thought into how we can continue to drive innovation and quality in medical education," he stated, "and came to the conclusion that ultrasound will play an integral role in the future of medicine." Because of this, he explained, in addition to the new white coats, each student would receive their own personal handheld ultrasound device. This was the first medical school in the nation to provide such a remarkable gift to its incoming students, a trend that has since continued at Nevada's Touro College of Osteopathic Medicine,[248] and most recently at Temple University School of Medicine.[249] "We don't want the education we give our ... medical students to be obsolete on the day that they graduate," explained Temple's interim dean Dr. Amy Goldberg, "we need to make sure that we are well ahead of the curve."[250]

Starting from Scratch

When Dr. Chris Fox was finishing his emergency medicine training, he was looking for a niche to focus on. One of his mentors recommended looking into ultrasound which "could be the future." At that time there were only two other emergency medicine ultrasound fellows in the country, and Fox became the third. "That wise piece of advice completely changed my life. I was just following career advice, but then I became really obsessed with it. It became my identity, that I could pick up a probe and look straight through someone's skin. I felt like I had a new superpower."[251] It's so hard to be a great doctor these days, he explained, with insurance headaches or administrative tasks, "but when you boil away the supernatant it comes down to me, my patient, and my probe. In that moment I'm having so much of a better doctor-patient interaction, and I think that's what keeps bringing me back to it. To this day it has made the practice of medicine so much more joyful. But it is hard to do, it took me a whole year of fellowship to really get good at it."

Dr. Fox (Figure 17) became an expert in point-of-care ultrasound and started his own educational company, traveling around the country for a decade, teaching a 2-day POCUS course to physicians and clinicians in all 49 states. "I'd go into a little town somewhere and teach 18 doctors, some trauma surgeons, some intensivists, mostly ER docs. It was a great experience. I got to travel around the country and get paid to teach. But in the end, I asked myself: could those people really do what I could do with it after 2 days? No. It was more like *this is what it can do*, and now it is up to you to come in on your days off and practice with it, and show those images to someone who knows what they are looking at. That's where I realized it was falling apart and started to think about medical students, and how we have four years with them."

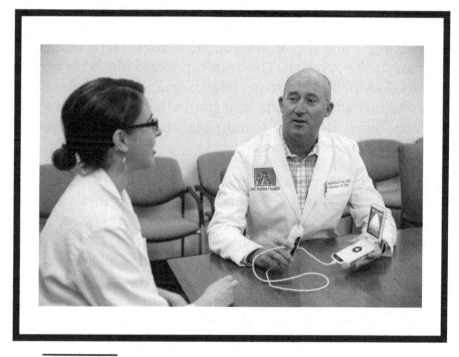

FIGURE 17 Dr. Chris Fox, a POCUS pioneer, Chair of Emergency Medicine, and director of ultrasound in medical education at UC Irvine. He developed one of the first comprehensive medical school POCUS curriculums.

Used with permission from Dr. Fox

He was already teaching a month-long elective for fourth-year medical students, so he wondered, "why not start with the first year, with anatomy and physiology?" He spoke with the deans of anatomy and physiology who loved the concept. Fox's plan was building steam but he needed more resources to help teach and roll it out, so he set up a meeting with the dean of the medical school. He brought the ultrasound machine to the meeting, along with a medical student that he used as a model. Dr. Fox had the student lay down and take his shirt off. "It was super awkward initially. The dean is a urologist so I'm ultrasounding the kidneys and the bladder. The dean takes the probe and starts scanning. He stares at the kidney and doesn't say much, then looks at the bladder and does the same." The meeting ended anticlimactically, but five days later Fox received a long e-mail from the dean expressing his excitement and recommending a follow up meeting to discuss the huge opportunities POCUS offered for their medical education. The dean connected him with various donors that enabled Fox to develop an extensive ultrasound curriculum, hire sonographers, and train other physician teachers to create what is now a sustainable, state-of-the-art medical school ultrasound curriculum.

In terms of his own clinical practice, as his POCUS skills developed he lost faith in the stethoscope and X-rays completely. "The more ultrasound I do, the more I realize how the X-ray is just as misleading as the stethoscope is. In general, I do not trust the negative predictive values of X-rays, and would never say a patient doesn't have an infiltrate based on a negative chest X-ray." As for the stethoscope, he feels there is still some value in asthmatic patients, but otherwise he uses ultrasound instead because the stethoscope "is just not that useful."

Despite all his clinical success with point-of-care ultrasound, what Dr. Fox seems most proud of is how ultrasound has improved the experience and medical knowledge of his students. He recalled a recent case of a 50-year-old male patient who had a syncopal episode. A visiting medical student was seeing the patient with him, and had her first *PO-kiss* very early in her career.

"She had recently learned aortic ultrasound and came across a huge aortic dissection. That finding completely redirected this person's care and they went to the operating room that evening," despite the fact that the patient was sitting in bed comfortably, not having chest pain. "Your student just totally saved someone's life today!" he wrote in an excited email to the visiting student's dean. Here was a clear example of how important and powerful POCUS can be, validating his mission to train medical students and expand their physical exam capabilities.

Similar to Fox, Dr. Soni is now the leader of point-of-care ultrasound training at UT San Antonio and the VA health care system. He spends much of his time training clinicians and formalizing training for internists. Along with other POCUS-wielding clinicians, he created a certification process through the national societies for doctors, nurse practitioners, and physician assistants hoping to become skilled with POCUS and have the confidence and ability to use it in everyday practice.[252] At this point, Soni feels the largest barriers to wider adoption are lack of training and time scarcity. Many clinicians "don't have time in their day to get trained or learn how to incorporate POCUS. So the question comes down to how do we give people bandwidth to incorporate new technologies that can improve care? Because there is obviously somewhat of a learning curve ... but the system we're locked into currently is based on encounters and numbers and many clinicians are pushed to run around as fast as they can and do a cursory evaluation of patients rather than take a more in-depth look with POCUS."

While significant barriers to wide adoption still remain, the increasing focus on ultrasound education in medical schools and residencies is a promising trend. Whether in primary care, urgent care, critical care, or in the hands of a specialist, point-of-care ultrasound offers a wide variety of enhancements to our clinical exam that we have only just begun to appreciate.

Science Fiction Becomes Science Non-fiction

In a 1968 episode of *Star Trek*, Captain Kirk is kidnapped by humanoid aliens, tortured unrelentingly, and shackled to the ceiling by his wrists. Science officer Spock and Dr. McCoy find him disheveled and minimally responsive. They release him from the chains and set him on a nearby table for examination. Dr. McCoy urgently takes out his medical tricorder, a device that can check organ function and detect disease with a wave of its detachable probe. He hovers it just above Captain Kirk's chest and within seconds he notes "severe heart damage, signs of congestion in both lungs," and "evidence of massive circulatory collapse."[253] This scene was featured in a YouTube video from 2009,[254] which cuts to the video's narrator discussing this "powerful, compact medical scanner," that has been a key tool for the science fiction doctors of *Star Trek*. "I should think the tricorder will be a real thing in the future," explained actor Alexander Siddig who played the character, Dr. Julian Bashir, in the early 1990s. "A diagnostic device which is really based on scanning. How on earth they are going to do that is for them to work out." That episode aired just three years after Dr. Feigenbaum figured out how to visualize a pericardial effusion with ultrasound, at a time when the only way to diagnose thoracic disease at the bedside was still with Laennec's stethoscope and the field of auscultation he pioneered.

In retrospect, the name "stethoscope" has garnered much confusion. Many viewed it as a misnomer since 'scope' translates to "an instrument for seeing,"[255] rather than hearing. As one doctor put it in the *Journal of the American Medical Association* in 1913: "the name of instruments by the use of which we see, when the proper terminology is used, end in the suffix "scope." While the name of instruments by which we hear should end in the suffix "phone." ... We may find ourselves reluctant to give up an error which can soon celebrate its centennial, but if a stethophone it is, why then miscall it?"[256]

Perhaps Laennec did not "miscall" it but rather named it for the aspirations he held for his beloved diagnostic tool; for what he envisioned could one day become of a handheld device at the bedside, a "means for enabling us to ascertain the character, not only of the action of the heart," as he described it, but also "the motion of all the thoracic viscera."[1] Maybe the stethoscope was named with the hope it would one day become the exemplification of what Dr. Forbes called "the wish of the ancient philosophers," to place "a window in the breast through which we can see the precise state of things within." If that is in fact the case, then point-of-care ultrasound, sometimes referred to as the sonoscope or the visual stethoscope, is the realization of Laennec's dream. The materialization of his audacious goal to see the inner workings of the thorax in real-time, not a technophile's distraction from our medical traditions.

POCUS is the natural progression of what Laennec started over 200 years ago, a tool he would undoubtedly add to his diagnostic repertoire were he able to, as he did with Auenbrugger's percussion or Hippocrates's succussion. It is a non-fiction device of today that was a science-fiction device of the 1960s, a handheld scanner that enables us all to be modern-day Dr. McCoys and instantly diagnose disease. Such incredible technology is the culmination of the underlying science and clinical techniques coupled with the innovative companies that enabled their bedside deployment.

Lichtenstein, Edler, Roelandt, Feigenbaum, and many others pushed diagnostic medicine into the *POCUS Era*, despite objections from the protectionists seeking to maintain the status quo. Through their determination to improve patient care with better diagnostics, propelled by companies like the Butterfly Network,[257] Vave Health,[258] Clarius,[259] or Sonosite,[260] a clinician can quickly diagnose disease with the modern-day tricorder in their white coat pocket.

When we look to the future of our bedside diagnostic capabilities, there are two divergent paths that emerge as our collective medical community contemplates what role - if any - that POCUS should play in our modern physical exam. One is the standard trajectory, driven by auditory inference through an analog listening device. It is comfortable. It is based on centuries of tradition, and it involves our most iconic tool. The alternative path is a challenging and uncomfortable one that requires extra training and a new way of thinking. It is one that endows clinicians with a superpower to peer through the body's walls and rule in or out disease with no ionizing radiation. It is a path that features a handheld head-to-toe imaging device that can diagnose blood clots and scan abdomens in outer space,[261-263] or function as full-body radiology departments in remote portions of Africa.[264] This path employs a device that is the epitome of what science fiction writer Arthur C. Clarke called "sufficiently advanced technology indistinguishable from magic," and it is a path that decreasingly relies on a stethoscope to detect the spectrum of audible noise our aging doctor-ears increasingly cannot discern.

If we yearn for an inspiring future of bedside diagnostic medicine, it is time to embrace this discomfort and take the latter path in lieu of fanning the flames of what little stethoscopic embers remain. Inspection, palpation, percussion, and auscultation have comprised the four pillars of our physical exam for over 200 years. Now, in the face of overwhelming evidence of improved diagnostic accuracy and patient care, it is time we embrace this new technique and make point-of-care ultrasound the fifth.

Acknowledgements

I want to thank my wife, daughter, and parents for their amazing support, ideas, and proofreading efforts. I want to thank my cousin and my brother and sister-in-law for reading drafts and offering valuable insight. I also want to thank my in-laws, my brother-in-law, my colleagues and friends for offering their detailed edits and honest feedback. I'd also like to thank the clinicians around the world who gave their unbridled opinions that enabled me to improve the final drafts. Lastly, I want to thank *you*, the reader, for taking the time to read it.

The medical history of our physical exam is vast and expansive, spanning multiple centuries, and is far more complex and nuanced than I was able to portray in this short text. I am passionate about POCUS and how it can change the medical diagnostics landscape, and am therefore biased in that regard. I made every attempt to present the evidence for the traditional physical exam and POCUS as fairly as possible, but I undoubtedly fell short in some areas. Despite many dozens of proof-reads and re-reads, there will likely be errors of omission or commission, but I assure you they were not made with haste.

If you enjoyed this book, if it challenged your preconceived notions or encouraged you to start using point-of-care ultrasound, please consider writing a review on Amazon and explaining what you liked most.

LITERATURE CITED

1. Laennec RTH, Forbes SJ. *A Treatise on the Diseases of the Chest, and on Mediate Auscultation.* S.S. and W. Wood; 1838.
2. Walker HK. The Origins of the History and Physical Examination. In: Walker HK, Hall WD, Hurst JW, eds. *Clinical Methods: The History, Physical, and Laboratory Examinations.* 3rd ed. Butterworths; 1990. Accessed May 15, 2021. http://www.ncbi.nlm.nih.gov/books/NBK458/
3. Jarcho S. Auenbrugger, Laennec, And John Keats: Some Notes on the Early History of Percussion and Auscultation. *Med Hist.* 1961;5(2):167-172.
4. Bedford DE. Auenbrugger's contribution to cardiology. History of percussion of the heart. *Br Heart J.* 1971;33(6):817-821.
5. McCarthy OR. Getting a feel for percussion. Published online 1999:8.
6. Stokes W. *An Introduction to the Use of the Stethoscope.* Dabor Science Publications; 1825.
7. Tomos I, Karakatsani A, Manali ED, Papiris SA. Celebrating Two Centuries since the Invention of the Stethoscope. René Théophile Hyacinthe Laënnec (1781–1826). *Ann Am Thorac Soc.* 2016;13(10):1667-1670. doi:10.1513/AnnalsATS.201605-411PS
8. Roguin A. Rene Theophile Hyacinthe Laennec (1781-1826): The Man Behind the Stethoscope. *Clin Med Res.* 2006;4(3):230-235. doi:10.3121/cmr.4.3.230
9. Montinari MR, Minelli S. The first 200 years of cardiac auscultation and future perspectives. *J Multidiscip Healthc.* 2019;12:183-189. doi:10.2147/JMDH.S193904
10. *The Cyclopaedia of Practical Medicine: Comprising Treatises on the Nature and Treatment of Disease, Materia Medica and Therapeutics, Medical Jurisprudence, Etc. Etc. Sof - Yaw, Supplement.* Sherwood, Gilbert, and Piper; 1835.
11. Hanna IR, Silverman ME. A history of cardiac auscultation and some of its contributors. *Am J Cardiol.* 2002;90(3):259-267.

doi:10.1016/S0002-9149(02)02465-7

12. Original cases, with dissections and observations. Books Published This Day. *The Morning Chronicle.* https://www.newspapers.com/image/?clipping_id=74551498&fcfToken=eyJhbGciOiJIUzI1NiIsInR5cCI6IkpXVCJ9.eyJmcmVlLXZpZXct aWQiOjM5MjEwNTUxMSSwiaWF0IjoxNjIxMjgxMzY5LCJleHAiOjE2MjEzNjc3Njl9.iqvZXHmEdIoRmyGkgxy-iSqVQifXFyZDl7eFayHSOcss. Published August 13, 1824.

13. Stallard v. Peacock. Special Jury. *Berrow's Worcester Journal.* https://www.newspapers.com/image/?clipping_id= 74546260&fcfToken=eyJhbGciOiJIUzI1NiIsInR5cCI6IkpXVCJ9.eyJmcmVlLXZpZXctaWQiOjQwMDk3Mzk3OC-wiaWF0IjoxNjIxMzMzOTYwLCJleHAiOjE2MjE0MjAzNjB9.7ukGpwCwYvLwqcL1O-0Z-E7NH0MAv8ebhGbi99hc2Rs. Published March 19, 1835.

14. Fox, Francis. Stethoscope with Elastic Ends. *The Derby Mercury.* https://www.newspapers.com/image/?clipping_id= 74545958&fcfToken=eyJhbGciOiJIUzI1NiIsInR5cCI6IkpXVCJ9.eyJmcmVlLXZpZXctaWQiOjM5MDY-wOTc3NiwiaWF0IjoxNjIxMzM5NTEwLCJleHAiOjE2MjEOMjU5MTB9.Er2dPL6qWqEocOqijFC2A_elQUaH1xIPXmbkyDO-JaI8. Published January 13, 1830.

15. Flint A. *Physical Exploration and Diagnosis of Diseases Affecting the Respiratory Organs.* Blanchard and Lea; 1856.

16. Stethoscope History | Littmann Stethoscopes | 3M United States. Accessed May 18, 2021. https://www.littmann.com/3M/en_US/littmann-stethoscopes/education-center/history/

17. Paxton S, Peckham M, Knibbs A. The Leeds Histology Guide. Published online 2003. Accessed September 30, 2021. https://www.histology.leeds.ac.uk/circulatory/capillaries.php

18. Hope J. *A Treatise on the Diseases of the Heart and Great Vessels.*; 1839.

19. Jackson SL, Tong X, King RJ, Loustalot F, Hong Y, Ritchey MD. National Burden of Heart Failure Events in the United States, 2006 to 2014. *Circ Heart Fail.* 2018;11(12):e004873. doi:10.1161/CIRCHEARTFAILURE.117.004873

20. Faustinella F, Jacobs RJ. The decline of clinical skills: a challenge for medical schools. *Int J Med Educ.* 2018;9:195-197. doi:10.5116/ijme.5b3f.9fb3

21. Obuchowski NA, Graham RJ, Baker ME, Powell KA. Ten Criteria for Effective Screening. Published online 2001:11.

22. Torino C, Gargani L, Sicari R, et al. The Agreement between Auscultation and Lung Ultrasound in Hemodialysis Patients: The LUST Study. *Clin J Am Soc Nephrol CJASN.* 2016;11(11):2005-2011. doi:10.2215/CJN.03890416

23. Dao Q, Krishnaswamy P, Kazanegra R, et al. Utility of B-type natriuretic peptide in the diagnosis of congestive heart failure in an urgent-care setting. *J Am Coll Cardiol.* 2001;37(2):379-385. doi:10.1016/S0735-1097(00)01156-6

24. Lichtenstein D, Grenier P. Comparative Diagnostic Performances of Auscultation, Chest Radiography, and Lung Ultrasonography in Acute Respiratory Distress Syndrome. 2004;100(1):7.

25. Pancaldi F, Sebastiani M, Cassone G, et al. Analysis of pulmonary sounds for the diagnosis of interstitial lung diseases secondary to rheumatoid arthritis. *Comput Biol Med.* 2018;96:91-97. doi:10.1016/j.compbiomed.2018.03.006

26. Kataoka H, Matsuno O. Age-Related Pulmonary Crackles (Rales) in Asymptomatic Cardiovascular Patients. *Ann Fam Med.* 2008;6(3):239-245. doi:10.1370/afm.834

27. Arts L, Lim EHT, van de Ven PM, Heunks L, Tuinman PR. The diagnostic accuracy of lung auscultation in adult patients with acute pulmonary pathologies: a meta-analysis. *Sci Rep.* 2020;10(1):7347. doi:10.1038/s41598-020-64405-6

28. Shine Music. *Whole Body Ultrasound Centered on the Lung A Holistic Approach by Daniel Lichtenstein.*; 2019. Accessed June 3, 2021. https://www.youtube.com/watch?v=RGIGdeAd-yU

29. Lichtenstein DA. E-mail Correspondence with Dr. Lichtenstein. Published online July 1, 2021.

30. sound | Origin and meaning of sound by Online Etymology Dictionary. Accessed May 31, 2021. https://www.etymonline.com/word/sound

31. Wiley TL, Chappell R, Carmichael L, Nondahl DM, Cruickshanks KJ. Changes in Hearing Thresholds over 10 Years in Older Adults. *J Am Acad Audiol.* 2008;19(4):281-371.

32. Point of Care Ultrasound - 2nd Edition. Accessed May 31, 2021. https://www.elsevier.com/books/point-of-care-ultrasound/soni/978-0-323-54470-2

33. Man who is blind can see like a bat. *BBC News.* https://www.bbc.com/news/av/magazine-35545476. Accessed May 31, 2021.

34. Basile V, Di Mauro A, Scalini E, et al. Lung ultrasound: a useful tool in diagnosis and management of bronchiolitis. *BMC Pediatr.* 2015;15(1):63. doi:10.1186/s12887-015-0380-1

35. Mahabadi N, Goizueta AA, Bordoni B. Anatomy, Thorax, Lung Pleura And Mediastinum. In: *StatPearls*. StatPearls Publishing; 2021. Accessed May 31, 2021. http://www.ncbi.nlm.nih.gov/books/NBK519048/

36. Rantanen NW. Diseases of the Thorax. *Vet Clin North Am Equine Pract.* 1986;2(1):49-66. doi:10.1016/S0749-0739(17)30732-0

37. K W, M G, Pe P, J H. Pneumothorax: evaluation by ultrasound--preliminary results. *J Thorac Imaging.* 1987;2(2):76-78.

38. Lichtenstein DA, Menu Y. A Bedside Ultrasound Sign Ruling Out Pneumothorax in the Critically Ill. *Chest.* 1995;108(5):1345-1348. doi:10.1378/chest.108.5.1345

39. de Lassence A, Timsit J-F, Tafflet M, et al. Pneumothorax in the intensive care unit: incidence, risk factors, and outcome. *Anesthesiology.* 2006;104(1):5-13. doi:10.1097/00000542-200601000-00003

40. Wilkerson RG, Stone MB. Sensitivity of Bedside Ultrasound and Supine Anteroposterior Chest Radiographs for the Identification of Pneumothorax After Blunt Trauma. *Acad Emerg Med.* 2010;17(1):11-17. doi:https://doi.org/10.1111/j.1553-2712.2009.00628.x

41. US EPA O. How much radiation am I exposed to when I have a CT scan? US EPA. Published February 11, 2019. Accessed May 30, 2021. https://www.epa.gov/radiation/how-much-radiation-am-i-exposed-when-i-have-ct-scan

42. Neff MA, Monk JSJ, Peters K, Nikhilesh A. Detection of Occult Pneumothoraces on Abdominal Computed Tomographic Scans in Trauma Patients. *J Trauma Acute Care Surg.* 2000;49(2):281-285.

43. Lichtenstein D, Mezière G, Biderman P, Gepner A. The "lung point": an ultrasound sign specific to pneumothorax. *Intensive Care Med.* 2000;26(10):1434-1440. doi:10.1007/s001340000627

44. Lichtenstein DA. *Whole Body Ultrasonography in the Critically Ill.* Springer Berlin Heidelberg; 2010. doi:10.1007/978-3-642-05328-3

45. Ding W, Shen Y, Yang J, He X, Zhang M. Diagnosis of Pneumothorax by Radiography and Ultrasonography. *Chest.* 2011;140(4):859-866. doi:10.1378/chest.10-2946

46. Alrajhi K, Woo MY, Vaillancourt C. Test Characteristics of Ultrasonography for the Detection of Pneumothorax. *Chest.* 2012;141(3):703-708. doi:10.1378/chest.11-0131

47. Alrajab S, Youssef AM, Akkus NI, Caldito G. Pleural ultrasonography versus chest radiography for the diagnosis of pneumothorax: review of the literature and meta-analysis. *Crit Care.* 2013;17(5):R208. doi:10.1186/cc13016

48. skullsinthestars. Infinity is weird... even in infinity mirrors! Skulls in the Stars. Published July 30, 2011. Accessed May 23, 2021. https://skullsinthestars.com/2011/07/30/infinity-is-weird-even-in-infinity-mirrors/

49. Lichtenstein D, Mezière G. A lung ultrasound sign allowing bedside distinction between pulmonary edema and COPD: the comet-tail artifact. *Intensive Care Med.* 1998;24(12):1331-1334. doi:10.1007/s001340050771

50. Ziskin MC, Thickman DI, Goldenberg NJ, Lapayowker MS, Becker JM. The comet tail artifact. *J Ultrasound Med.* 1982;1(1):1-7. doi:https://doi.org/10.7863/jum.1982.1.1.1

51. Lichtenstein D, Mézière G, Biderman P, Gepner A, Barré O. The Comet-tail Artifact: An Ultrasound Sign of Alveolar-Interstitial Syndrome. *Am J Respir Crit Care Med.* 1997;156(5):1640-1646. doi:10.1164/ajrccm.156.5.96-07096

52. Lichtenstein DA. *Lung Ultrasound in the Critically Ill: The BLUE Protocol.* Springer International Publishing; 2016. doi:10.1007/978-3-319-15371-1

53. Ochs M, Nyengaard JR, Jung A, et al. The Number of Alveoli in the Human Lung. *Am J Respir Crit Care Med.* 2004;169(1):120-124. doi:10.1164/rccm.200308-1107OC

54. American Lung Association. How Your Lungs Get the Job Done. Accessed September 30, 2021. https://www.lung.org/blog/how-your-lungs-work

55. Jozwiak M, Teboul J-L, Monnet X. Extravascular lung water in critical care: recent advances and clinical applications. *Ann Intensive Care.* 2015;5(1):38. doi:10.1186/s13613-015-0081-9

56. Osler SW. *The Principles and Practice of Medicine.* D. Appleton and company; 1920.

57. Agricola E, Bove T, Oppizzi M, et al. "Ultrasound Comet-Tail Images": A Marker Of Pulmonary Edema: A Comparative Study With Wedge Pressure And Extravascular Lung Water. *Chest.* 2005;127(5):1690-1695. doi:10.1378/chest.127.5.1690

58. Frassi F, Gargani L, Gligorova S, Ciampi Q, Mottola G, Picano E. Clinical and echocardiographic determinants of ultrasound lung comets. *Eur J Echocardiogr J Work Group Echocardiogr Eur Soc Cardiol.* 2007;8(6):474-479. doi:10.1016/j.euje.2006.09.004

59. Volpicelli G, Caramello V, Cardinale L, Mussa A, Bar F, Frascisco MF. Bedside ultrasound of the lung for the monitoring of acute decompensated heart failure. *Am J Emerg Med.* 2008;26(5):585-591. doi:10.1016/j.ajem.2007.09.014

60. Mallamaci F, Benedetto FA, Tripepi R, et al. Detection of Pulmonary Congestion by Chest Ultrasound in Dialysis Patients. *JACC Cardiovasc Imaging.* 2010;3(6):586-594. doi:10.1016/j.jcmg.2010.02.005

61. Noble VE, Murray AF, Capp R, Sylvia-Reardon MH, Steele DJR, Liteplo A. Ultrasound Assessment for Extravascular Lung Water in Patients Undergoing Hemodialysis: Time Course for Resolution. *Chest.* 2009;135(6):1433-1439. doi:10.1378/chest.08-1811

62. Nakao S, Vaillancourt C, Taljaard M, Nemnom M-J, Woo MY, Stiell IG. Diagnostic Accuracy of Lung Point-Of-Care Ultrasonography for Acute Heart Failure Compared With Chest X-Ray Study Among Dyspneic Older Patients in the Emergency Department. *J Emerg Med.* Published online March 29, 2021. doi:10.1016/j.jemermed.2021.02.019

63. Cibinel GA, Casoli G, Elia F, et al. Diagnostic accuracy and reproducibility of pleural and lung ultrasound in discriminating cardiogenic causes of acute dyspnea in the Emergency Department. *Intern Emerg Med.* 2012;7(1):65-70. doi:10.1007/s11739-011-0709-1

64. Prosen G, Klemen P, Strnad M, Grmec Š. Combination of lung ultrasound (a comet-tail sign) and N-terminal pro-brain natriuretic peptide in differentiating acute heart failure from chronic obstructive pulmonary disease and asthma as cause of acute dyspnea in prehospital emergency setting. *Crit Care.* 2011;15(2):R114. doi:10.1186/cc10140

65. Pivetta E, Goffi A, Lupia E, et al. Lung Ultrasound-Implemented Diagnosis of Acute Decompensated Heart Failure in the ED. *Chest.* 2015;148(1):202-210. doi:10.1378/chest.14-2608

66. Wang Y, Shen Z, Lu X, Zhen Y, Li H. Sensitivity and specificity of ultrasound for the diagnosis of acute pulmonary edema: a systematic review and meta-analysis. *Med Ultrason.* 2018;1(1):32-36. doi:10.11152/mu-1223

67. Al Deeb M, Barbic S, Featherstone R, Dankoff J, Barbic D. Point-of-care ultrasonography for the diagnosis of acute cardiogenic pulmonary edema in patients presenting with acute dyspnea: a systematic review and meta-analysis. *Acad Emerg Med Off J Soc Acad Emerg Med.* 2014;21(8):843-852. doi:10.1111/acem.12435

68. Maw AM, Hassanin A, Ho PM, et al. Diagnostic Accuracy of Point-of-Care Lung Ultrasonography and Chest Radiography in Adults With Symptoms Suggestive of Acute Decompensated Heart Failure. *JAMA Netw Open.* 2019;2(3). doi:10.1001/jamanetworkopen.2019.0703

69. Lichtenstein DA, Lascols N, Mezière G, Gepner A. Ultrasound diagnosis of alveolar consolidation in the critically ill. *Intensive Care Med.* 2004;30(2):276-281. doi:10.1007/s00134-003-2075-6

70. Hayden GE, Wrenn KW. Chest Radiograph vs. Computed Tomography Scan in the Evaluation for Pneumonia. *J Emerg Med.* 2009;36(3):266-270. doi:10.1016/j.jemermed.2007.11.042

71. Heussel CP, Kauczor H-U, Heussel GE, et al. Pneumonia in Febrile Neutropenic Patients and in Bone Marrow and Blood Stem-Cell Transplant Recipients: Use of High-Resolution Computed Tomography. *J Clin Oncol.* 1999;17(3):796-796. doi:10.1200/JCO.1999.17.3.796

72. Self WH, Courtney DM, McNaughton CD, Wunderink RG, Kline JA. High Discordance of Chest X-ray and CT for Detection of Pulmonary Opacities in ED Patients: Implications for Diagnosing Pneumonia. *Am J Emerg Med.* 2013;31(2):401-405. doi:10.1016/j.ajem.2012.08.041

73. Edwards RM, Godwin JD, Hippe DS, Kicska G. A Quantitative Approach to Distinguish Pneumonia From Atelectasis Using Computed Tomography Attenuation. *J Comput Assist Tomogr.* 2016;40(5):746-751. doi:10.1097/RCT.0000000000000438

74. Lichtenstein D, Mezière G, Seitz J. The Dynamic Air Bronchogram: A Lung Ultrasound Sign of Alveolar Consolidation Ruling Out Atelectasis. *CHEST.* 2009;135(6):1421-1425. doi:10.1378/chest.08-2281

75. Tierney DM, Huelster JS, Overgaard JD, et al. Comparative Performance of Pulmonary Ultrasound, Chest Radiograph, and CT Among Patients With Acute Respiratory Failure. *Crit Care Med.* 2020;48(2):151-157. doi:10.1097/CCM.0000000000004124

76. Liu X, Lian R, Tao Y, Gu C, Zhang G. Lung ultrasonography: an effective way to diagnose community-acquired pneumonia. *Emerg Med J.* 2015;32(6):433-438. doi:10.1136/emermed-2013-203039

77. Claes A-S, Clapuyt P, Menten R, Michoux N, Dumitriu D. Performance of chest ultrasound in pediatric pneumonia. *Eur J Radiol.* 2017;88:82-87. doi:10.1016/j.ejrad.2016.12.032

78. Gao Y-Q, Qiu R-X, Liu J, Zhang L, Ren X-L, Qin S-J. Lung ultrasound completely replaced chest X-ray for diagnosing neonatal lung diseases: a 3-year clinical practice report from a neonatal intensive care unit in China. *J Matern Fetal Neonatal Med.* 2020;0(0):1-8. doi:10.1080/14767058.2020.1830369

79. Xirouchaki N, Magkanas E, Vaporidi K, et al. Lung ultrasound in critically ill patients: comparison with bedside chest radiography. *Intensive Care Med.* 2011;37(9):1488-1493. doi:10.1007/s00134-011-2317-y

80. Pare J, Camelo I, Mayo K, et al. Point-of-care Lung Ultrasound Is More Sensitive than Chest Radiograph for Evaluation of COVID-19. *West J Emerg Med.* 2020;21(4). doi:10.5811/westjem.2020.5.47743

81. Amatya Y, Rupp J, Russell FM, Saunders J, Bales B, House DR. Diagnostic use of lung ultrasound compared to chest radiograph for suspected pneumonia in a resource-limited setting. *Int J Emerg Med.* 2018;11(1):8. doi:10.1186/s12245-018-0170-2

82. Alzahrani SA, Al-Salamah MA, Al-Madani WH, Elbarbary MA. Systematic review and meta-analysis for the use of ultrasound versus radiology in diagnosing of pneumonia. *Crit Ultrasound J.* 2017;9(1):6. doi:10.1186/s13089-017-0059-y

83. Balk DS, Lee C, Schafer J, et al. Lung ultrasound compared to chest X-ray for diagnosis of pediatric pneumonia: A meta-analysis. *Pediatr Pulmonol.* 2018;53(8):1130-1139. doi:https://doi.org/10.1002/ppul.24020

84. Llor C, Bjerrum L. Antimicrobial resistance: risk associated with antibiotic overuse and initiatives to reduce the problem. *Ther Adv Drug Saf.* 2014;5(6):229-241. doi:10.1177/2042098614554919

85. Wong CL. Does This Patient Have a Pleural Effusion? *JAMA.* 2009;301(3):309. doi:10.1001/jama.2008.937

86. Soni NJ, Franco R, Velez MI, et al. Ultrasound in the diagnosis and management of pleural effusions. *J Hosp Med.* 2015;10(12):811-816. doi:10.1002/jhm.2434

87. Gryminski J, Krakówka P, Lypacewicz G. The Diagnosis of Pleural Effusion by Ultrasonic and Radiologic Techniques. *Chest.* 1976;70(1):33-37. doi:10.1378/chest.70.1.33

88. Kalokairinou-Motogna M, Maratou K, Paianid I, et al. Application of color Doppler ultrasound in the study of small pleural effusion. *Med Ultrason.* 2010;12(1):12-16.

89. Kitazono MT, Lau CT, Parada AN, Renjen P, Miller WT.

Differentiation of Pleural Effusions From Parenchymal Opacities: Accuracy of Bedside Chest Radiography. *Am J Roentgenol.* 2010;194(2):407-412. doi:10.2214/AJR.09.2950

90. Brixey AG, Luo Y, Skouras V, Awdankiewicz A, Light RW. The efficacy of chest radiographs in detecting parapneumonic effusions. *Respirol Carlton Vic.* 2011;16(6):1000-1004. doi:10.1111/j.1440-1843.2011.02006.x

91. Lichtenstein D, Hulot J-S, Rabiller A, Tostivint I, Mezière G. Feasibility and safety of ultrasound-aided thoracentesis in mechanically ventilated patients. *Intensive Care Med.* 1999;25(9):955-958. doi:10.1007/s001340050988

92. Emamian SA, Kaasbøl M-A, Olsen JF, Pedersen JF. Accuracy of the diagnosis of pleural effusion on supine chest X-ray. *Eur Radiol.* 1997;7(1):57-60. doi:10.1007/s003300050109

93. Xirouchaki N, Kondili E, Prinianakis G, Malliotakis P, Georgopoulos D. Impact of lung ultrasound on clinical decision making in critically ill patients. *Intensive Care Med.* 2014;40(1):57-65. doi:10.1007/s00134-013-3133-3

94. Rocco M, Carbone I, Morelli A, et al. Diagnostic accuracy of bedside ultrasonography in the ICU: feasibility of detecting pulmonary effusion and lung contusion in patients on respiratory support after severe blunt thoracic trauma. *Acta Anaesthesiol Scand.* 2008;52(6):776-784. doi:10.1111/j.1399-6576.2008.01647.x

95. Kataoka H, Takada S. The role of thoracic ultrasonography for evaluation of patients with decompensated chronic heart failure. *J Am Coll Cardiol.* 2000;35(6):1638-1646. doi:10.1016/S0735-1097(00)00602-1

96. Lee FCY. The Curtain Sign in Lung Ultrasound. *J Med Ultrasound.* 2017;25(2):101-104. doi:10.1016/j.jmu.2017.04.005

97. Hart J. Cancer Mortality in Six Lowest Versus Six Highest Elevation Jurisdictions in the U.S. *Dose-Response.* 2010;9(1):50-58. doi:10.2203/dose-response.09-051.Hart

98. Radiation risk from medical imaging. Harvard Health. Published September 22, 2010. Accessed October 14, 2021. https://www.health.harvard.edu/cancer/radiation-risk-from-medical-imaging

99. Information for Radiation Workers. NRC Web. Accessed June 17, 2021. https://www.nrc.gov/about-nrc/radiation/health-effects/info.html

100. Sodickson A, Baeyens PF, Andriole KP, et al. Recurrent CT, Cumulative Radiation Exposure, and Associated Ra-

diation-induced Cancer Risks from CT of Adults. *Radiology.* 2009;251(1):175-184. doi:10.1148/radiol.2511081296

101. Lee CI, Haims AH, Monico EP, Brink JA, Forman HP. Diagnostic CT Scans: Assessment of Patient, Physician, and Radiologist Awareness of Radiation Dose and Possible Risks. *Radiology.* 2004;231(2):393-398. doi:10.1148/radiol.2312030767

102. Brenner DJ, Elliston CD, Hall EJ, Berdon WE. Estimated Risks of Radiation-Induced Fatal Cancer from Pediatric CT. *Am J Roentgenol.* 2001;176(2):289-296. doi:10.2214/ajr.176.2.1760289

103. Brenner DJ, Hall EJ. Computed Tomography — An Increasing Source of Radiation Exposure. *N Engl J Med.* 2007;357(22):2277-2284. doi:10.1056/NEJMra072149

104. Radiation Risks and Pediatric Computed Tomography - National Cancer Institute. Published August 20, 2002. Accessed June 12, 2021. https://www.cancer.gov/about-cancer/causes-prevention/risk/radiation/pediatric-ct-scans

105. Strauss KJ, Somasundaram E, Sengupta D, Marin JR, Brady SL. Radiation Dose for Pediatric CT: Comparison of Pediatric versus Adult Imaging Facilities. *Radiology.* 2019;291(1):158-167. doi:10.1148/radiol.2019181753

106. Yu C-C. Radiation Safety in the Neonatal Intensive Care Unit: Too Little or Too Much Concern? *Pediatr Neonatol.* 2010;51(6):311-319. doi:10.1016/S1875-9572(10)60061-7

107. Lichtenstein DA, Mezière GA. Relevance of lung ultrasound in the diagnosis of acute respiratory failure: the BLUE protocol. *Chest.* 2008;134(1):117-125. doi:10.1378/chest.07-2800

108. Lichtenstein D. Novel approaches to ultrasonography of the lung and pleural space: where are we now? *Breathe.* 2017;13(2):100-111. doi:10.1183/20734735.004717

109. Volpicelli G, Elbarbary M, Blaivas M, et al. International evidence-based recommendations for point-of-care lung ultrasound. *Intensive Care Med.* 2012;38(4):577-591. doi:10.1007/s00134-012-2513-4

110. Kobal SL, Trento L, Baharami S, et al. Comparison of Effectiveness of Hand-Carried Ultrasound to Bedside Cardiovascular Physical Examination. *Am J Cardiol.* 2005;96(7):1002-1006. doi:10.1016/j.amjcard.2005.05.060

111. Levine H. Rest Heart Rate and Life Expectancy. doi:10.1016/S0735-1097(97)00246-5

112. Harvey W, Willis R, Society S. *The Works of William Harvey ...* Sydenham Society; 1847.

113. Fulton A. *Memoir of the Late James Hope, M.D.* Hatchard; 1842.

114. Rackow E, Siiferman E. The James Hope Presentation Stethoscope. Accessed June 18, 2021. https://www.antiquemed.com/james_hope.htm

115. A Famous Cardiac Controversy. Accessed June 18, 2021. https://link.springer.com/content/pdf/10.1007/BF02954484.pdf

116. Evidence-Based Physical Diagnosis - 4th Edition. Accessed July 17, 2021. https://www.elsevier.com/books/evidence-based-physical-diagnosis/9780323392761

117. Flint A. A practical treatise on the diagnosis, pathology, and treatment of diseases of the heart. by Austin Flint: Good Hardcover (1859) First Edition. | Sequitur Books. Accessed September 26, 2021. https://www.abebooks.com/first-edition/practical-treatise-diagnosis-pathology-treatment-diseases/22666337343/bd

118. Clair EWS, Z. Oddone E, A. Waugh R, Ralph Corey G, R. Feussner J. Assessing Housestaff Diagnostic Skills Using a Cardiology Patient Simulator. *Ann Intern Med.* Published online March 10, 2020. Accessed July 17, 2021. https://www.acpjournals.org/doi/abs/10.7326/0003-4819-117-9-751

119. Mangione S, Nieman LZ. Cardiac Auscultatory Skills of Internal Medicine and Family Practice Trainees: A Comparison of Diagnostic Proficiency. *JAMA.* 1997;278(9):717-722. doi:10.1001/jama.1997.03550090041030

120. Kinney EL. Causes of false-negative auscultation of regurgitant lesions. *J Gen Intern Med.* 1988;3(5):429-434. doi:10.1007/BF02595918

121. Rahko PS. Prevalence of Regurgitant Murmurs in Patients with Valvular Regurgitation Detected by Doppler Echocardiography. *Ann Intern Med.* 1989;111(6):466-472. doi:10.7326/0003-4819-111-6-466

122. Attenhofer Jost CH, Turina J, Mayer K, et al. Echocardiography in the evaluation of systolic murmurs of unknown cause. *Am J Med.* 2000;108(8):614-620. doi:10.1016/S0002-9343(00)00361-2

123. Iversen KK, Teisner AS, Bay M, Kirk V, Boesgaard S, Nielsen H. Heart murmur and echocardiographic findings in 2,907 non-selected patients admitted to hospital. *Ugeskr Laeger.* 2006;168(26-32):2551-2554.

124. Gardezi SKM, Myerson SG, Chambers J, et al. Car-

diac auscultation poorly predicts the presence of valvular heart disease in asymptomatic primary care patients. *Heart.* 2018;104(22):1832-1835. doi:10.1136/heartjnl-2018-313082

125. Sztajzel JM, Picard-Kossovsky M, Lerch R, Vuille C, Sarasin FP. Accuracy of cardiac auscultation in the era of Doppler-echocardiography: A comparison between cardiologists and internists. *Int J Cardiol.* 2010;138(3):308-310. doi:10.1016/j.ijcard.2008.06.066

126. Roelandt JRTC. The decline of our physical examination skills: is echocardiography to blame? *Eur Heart J - Cardiovasc Imaging.* 2014;15(3):249-252. doi:10.1093/ehjci/jet195

127. Singh S, Goyal A. The Origin of Echocardiography. *Tex Heart Inst J.* 2007;34(4):431-438.

128. Nilsson J, Westling H. Ultrasound in Lund - three world premieres. *Clin Physiol Funct Imaging.* 2004;24(3):137-140. doi:10.1111/j.1475-097X.2004.00540.x

129. Feigenbaum H. Evolution of Echocardiography. *Circulation.* 1996;93(7):1321-1327. doi:10.1161/01.CIR.93.7.1321

130. Fraser AG. Inge Edler and the origins of clinical echocardiography. *Eur J Echocardiogr J Work Group Echocardiogr Eur Soc Cardiol.* 2001;2(1):3-5. doi:10.1053/euje.2001.0082

131. Feigenbaum MD H. Interview on Echo Origins. Published online August 31, 2021.

132. Maron BJ. Harvey Feigenbaum, MD, and the Creation of Clinical Echocardiography: A Conversation With Barry J. Maron, MD. *Am J Cardiol.* 2017;120(11):2085-2099. doi:10.1016/j.amjcard.2017.08.033

133. Feigenbaum H, Waldhausen JA, Hyde LP. Ultrasound Diagnosis of Pericardial Effusion. *JAMA.* 1965;191(9):711-714. doi:10.1001/jama.1965.03080090025006

134. ASE360. *Harvey Feigenbaum Talks About the Beginning of Echocardiography.* Accessed July 5, 2021. https://www.youtube.com/watch?v=QsM9nkbY12M&t=285s

135. Silverman ME. The Third Heart Sound. In: Walker HK, Hall WD, Hurst JW, eds. *Clinical Methods: The History, Physical, and Laboratory Examinations.* 3rd ed. Butterworths; 1990. Accessed July 10, 2021. http://www.ncbi.nlm.nih.gov/books/NBK342/

136. Tribouilloy CM, Enriquez-Sarano M, Mohty D, et al. Pathophysiologic determinants of third heart sounds: a prospective clinical and Doppler echocardiographic study. *Am J Med.* 2001;111(2):96-102. doi:10.1016/S0002-9343(01)00769-0

137. Butman Samuel M., Ewy Gordon A., Standen James R., Kern Karl B., Hahn Elizabeth. Bedside cardiovascular examination in patients with severe chronic heart failure: Importance of rest or inducible jugular venous distension. *J Am Coll Cardiol.* 1993;22(4):968-974. doi:10.1016/0735-1097(93)90405-P

138. Wang CS, FitzGerald JM, Schulzer M, Mak E, Ayas NT. Does This Dyspneic Patient in the Emergency Department Have Congestive Heart Failure? *JAMA.* 2005;294(15):1944-1956. doi:10.1001/jama.294.15.1944

139. Caldentey Guillem, Khairy Paul, Roy Denis, et al. Prognostic Value of the Physical Examination in Patients With Heart Failure and Atrial Fibrillation. *JACC Heart Fail.* 2014;2(1):15-23. doi:10.1016/j.jchf.2013.10.004

140. Ishmail AA, Wing S, Ferguson J, Hutchinson TA, Magder S, Flegel KM. Interobserver Agreement by Auscultation in the Presence of a Third Heart Sound in Patients with Congestive Heart Failure. *Chest.* 1987;91(6):870-873. doi:10.1378/chest.91.6.870

141. Lok CE, Morgan CD, Ranganathan N. The Accuracy and Interobserver Agreement in Detecting the 'Gallop Sounds' by Cardiac Auscultation. *Chest.* 1998;114(5):1283-1288. doi:10.1378/chest.114.5.1283

142. Melamed R, Sprenkle MD, Ulstad VK, Herzog CA, Leatherman JW. Assessment of Left Ventricular Function by Intensivists Using Hand-Held Echocardiography. *Chest.* 2009;135(6):1416-1420. doi:10.1378/chest.08-2440

143. Moore CL, Rose GA, Tayal VS, Sullivan DM, Arrowood JA, Kline JA. Determination of Left Ventricular Function by Emergency Physician Echocardiography of Hypotensive Patients. *Acad Emerg Med.* 2002;9(3):186-193. doi:10.1197/aemj.9.3.186

144. Massie BM, Schiller NB, Ratshin RA. Mitral-Septal Separation: New Echocardiographic Index of Left Ventricular Function. :9.

145. Siliv NS, Yamanoglu A, Pınar P, Yamanoglu NGC, Torlak F, Parlak I. Estimation of Cardiac Systolic Function Based on Mitral Valve Movements: An Accurate Bedside Tool for Emergency Physicians in Dyspneic Patients. *J Ultrasound Med.* 2019;38(4):1027-1038. doi:10.1002/jum.14791

146. Boon SC, Matta JEL, Kraemer CVE, Tuinman PR, van Westerloo DJ. POCUS series: E-point septal separation, a quick assessment of reduced left ventricular ejection fraction in a POCUS setting. 28(3):3.

147. Jenkins S, Alabed S, Swift A, et al. Diagnostic accuracy of

handheld cardiac ultrasound device for assessment of left ventricular structure and function: systematic review and meta-analysis. *Heart*. Published online August 6, 2021. doi:10.1136/heartjnl-2021-319561

148. Panoulas VF, Daigeler A-L, Malaweera ASN, et al. Pocket-size hand-held cardiac ultrasound as an adjunct to clinical examination in the hands of medical students and junior doctors. *Eur Heart J Cardiovasc Imaging*. 2013;14(4):323-330. doi:10.1093/ehjci/jes140

149. Spencer KT, Anderson AS, Bhargava A, et al. Physician-performed point-of-care echocardiography using a laptop platform compared with physical examination in the cardiovascular patient. *J Am Coll Cardiol*. 2001;37(8):2013-2018. doi:10.1016/S0735-1097(01)01288-8

150. Kaul S. Is it Time to Replace Physical Examination with a Hand-Held Ultrasound Device? *J Cardiovasc Echography*. 2014;24(4):97-102. doi:10.4103/2211-4122.147199

151. Mehta M, Jacobson T, Peters D, et al. Handheld Ultrasound Versus Physical Examination in Patients Referred for Transthoracic Echocardiography for a Suspected Cardiac Condition. *JACC Cardiovasc Imaging*. 2014;7(10):983-990. doi:10.1016/j.jcmg.2014.05.011

152. Brennan JM, Blair JE, Goonewardena S, et al. A Comparison by Medicine Residents of Physical Examination Versus Hand-Carried Ultrasound for Estimation of Right Atrial Pressure. *Am J Cardiol*. 2007;99(11):1614-1616. doi:10.1016/j.amjcard.2007.01.037

153. Stokke TM, Ruddox V, Sarvari SI, Otterstad JE, Aune E, Edvardsen T. Brief Group Training of Medical Students in Focused Cardiac Ultrasound May Improve Diagnostic Accuracy of Physical Examination. *J Am Soc Echocardiogr*. 2014;27(11):1238-1246. doi:10.1016/j.echo.2014.08.001

154. Martin LD, Howell EE, Ziegelstein RC, et al. Hand-carried Ultrasound Performed by Hospitalists: Does It Improve the Cardiac Physical Examination? *Am J Med*. 2009;122(1):35-41. doi:10.1016/j.amjmed.2008.07.022

155. Galderisi M, Santoro A, Versiero M, et al. Improved cardiovascular diagnostic accuracy by pocket size imaging device in non-cardiologic outpatients: the NaUSiCa (Naples Ultrasound Stethoscope in Cardiology) study. *Cardiovasc Ultrasound*. 2010;8(1):51. doi:10.1186/1476-7120-8-51

156. Bello VD, Carrubba SL, Conte L, et al. Incremental Value of Pocket-Sized Echocardiography in Addition to Physical Examination during Inpatient Cardiology Evaluation: A Multicenter Italian Study (SIEC). *Echocardiography*. 2015;32(10):1463-1470. doi:10.1111/echo.12910

157. DeCara JM, Kirkpatrick JN, Spencer KT, et al. Use of hand-carried ultrasound devices to augment the accuracy of medical student bedside cardiac diagnoses. *J Am Soc Echocardiogr*. 2005;18(3):257-263. doi:10.1016/j.echo.2004.11.015

158. KIMURA BJ, AMUNDSON SA, WILLIS CL, GILPIN EA, DEMARIA AN. Usefulness of a hand-held ultrasound device for bedside examination of left ventricular function. *Useful Hand-Held Ultrasound Device Bedside Exam Left Ventricular Funct*. 2002;90(9):1038-1039.

159. Cardim N, Fernandez Golfin C, Ferreira D, et al. Usefulness of a New Miniaturized Echocardiographic System in Outpatient Cardiology Consultations as an Extension of Physical Examination. *J Am Soc Echocardiogr*. 2011;24(2):117-124. doi:10.1016/j.echo.2010.09.017

160. Lewis T. Remarks on Early Signs of Cardiac Failure of The Congestive Type. *Br Med J*. 1930;1(3618):849-852.

161. LANCISI GM. *J. M. Lancisii … de motu cordis, et aneurysmatibus opus posthumum, etc.*; 1728.

162. CHIACO JMSC, PARIKH NI, FERGUSSON DJ. The jugular venous pressure revisited. *Cleve Clin J Med*. 2013;80(10):638-644. doi:10.3949/ccjm.80a.13039

163. Short DS. The Jugular Venous Pulse. *Postgrad Med J*. 1957;33(382):389-394.

164. Applefeld MM. The Jugular Venous Pressure and Pulse Contour. In: Walker HK, Hall WD, Hurst JW, eds. *Clinical Methods: The History, Physical, and Laboratory Examinations*. 3rd ed. Butterworths; 1990. Accessed August 12, 2021. http://www.ncbi.nlm.nih.gov/books/NBK300/

165. Davison R, Cannon R. Estimation of central venous pressure by examination of jugular veins. *Am Heart J*. 1974;87(3):279-282. doi:10.1016/0002-8703(74)90064-7

166. Connors AF, McCaffree DR, Gray BA. Evaluation of right-heart catheterization in the critically ill patient without acute myocardial infarction. *N Engl J Med*. 1983;308(5):263-267. doi:10.1056/NEJM198302033080508

167. Cook DJ. Clinical Assessment of Central Venous Pressure in the

Critically Ill. *Am J Med Sci.* 1990;299(3):175-178. doi:10.1097/00000441-199003000-00006

168. Pr E, As J, Dp S. Clinical evaluation compared to pulmonary artery catheterization in the hemodynamic assessment of critically ill patients. *Crit Care Med.* 1984;12(7):549-553. doi:10.1097/00003246-198407000-00001

169. Demeria DD, MacDougall A, Spurek M, et al. Comparison of Clinical Measurement of Jugular Venous Pressure Versus Measured Central Venous Pressure. *Chest.* 2004;126(4):747S. doi:10.1378/chest.126.4_MeetingAbstracts.747S

170. Sinisalo J, Rapola J, Rossinen J, Kupari M. Simplifying the Estimation of Jugular Venous Pressure. *Am J Cardiol.* 2007;100(12):1779-1781. doi:10.1016/j.amjcard.2007.07.030

171. McGee SR. Physical examination of venous pressure: A critical review. *Am Heart J.* 1998;136(1):10-18. doi:10.1016/S0002-8703(98)70175-9

172. Ogden CL, Fryar CD, Martin CB, et al. Trends in Obesity Prevalence by Race and Hispanic Origin—1999-2000 to 2017-2018. *JAMA.* 2020;324(12):1208. doi:10.1001/jama.2020.14590

173. Bloomfield RA, Lauson HD, Cournand A, Breed ES, Richards DW. Recording of Right Heart Pressures in Normal Subjects and in Patients with Chronic Pulmonary Disease and Various Types of Cardio-Circulatory Disease. *J Clin Invest.* 1946;25(4):639-664. doi:10.1172/JCI101746

174. Kovacs G, Avian A, Olschewski A, Olschewski H. Zero reference level for right heart catheterisation. *Eur Respir J.* 2013;42(6):1586-1594. doi:10.1183/09031936.00050713

175. Seth R, Magner P, Matzinger F, Walraven CV. How Far Is the Sternal Angle from the Mid-right Atrium? *J Gen Intern Med.* 2002;17(11):861-865. doi:https://doi.org/10.1046/j.1525-1497.2002.20101.x

176. Lipton B. Estimation of central venous pressure by ultrasound of the internal jugular vein. *Am J Emerg Med.* 2000;18(4):432-434. doi:10.1053/ajem.2000.7335

177. Beddy P, Geoghegan T, Ramesh N, et al. Valsalva and gravitational variability of the internal jugular vein and common femoral vein: Ultrasound assessment. *Eur J Radiol.* 2006;58(2):307-309. doi:10.1016/j.ejrad.2005.11.005

178. Simon MA, Kliner DE, Girod JP, Moguillansky D, Villanueva FS, Pacella JJ. Detection of elevated right atrial pressure using a simple bedside ultrasound measure. *Am Heart J.*

2010;159(3):421-427. doi:10.1016/j.ahj.2010.01.004

179. Donahue SP, Wood JP, Patel BM, Quinn JV. Correlation of sonographic measurements of the internal jugular vein with central venous pressure. *Am J Emerg Med.* 2009;27(7):851-855. doi:10.1016/j.ajem.2008.06.005

180. Deol GR, Collett N, Ashby A, Schmidt GA. Ultrasound Accurately Reflects the Jugular Venous Examination but Underestimates Central Venous Pressure. *Chest.* 2011;139(1):95-100. doi:10.1378/chest.10-1301

181. Siva B, Hunt A, Boudville N. The sensitivity and specificity of ultrasound estimation of central venous pressure using the internal jugular vein. *J Crit Care.* 2012;27(3):315.e7-315.e11. doi:10.1016/j.jcrc.2011.09.008

182. Hoeper MM, Lee SH, Voswinckel R, et al. Complications of Right Heart Catheterization Procedures in Patients With Pulmonary Hypertension in Experienced Centers. *J Am Coll Cardiol.* 2006;48(12):2546-2552. doi:10.1016/j.jacc.2006.07.061

183. Manda YR, Baradhi KM. Cardiac Catheterization Risks and Complications. In: *StatPearls.* StatPearls Publishing; 2021. Accessed June 26, 2021. http://www.ncbi.nlm.nih.gov/books/NBK531461/

184. New Method for Noninvasive Quantification of Central Venous Pressure by Ultrasound. doi:10.1161/CIRCIMAGING.114.003085

185. Istrail L, Stepanova M. *Novel Point-of-Care Ultrasound (POCUS) Technique to Modernize the JVP Exam and Rule out Elevated Right Atrial Pressures.*; 2021:2021.10.14.21264891. doi:10.1101/2021.10.14.21264891. Pre-print.

186. Kennedy JW, Baxley WA, Figley MM, Dodge HT, Blackmon JR. Quantitative Angiocardiography: The Normal Left Ventricle in Man. *Circulation.* 1966;34(2):272-278. doi:10.1161/01.CIR.34.2.272

187. Drazner MH, Hamilton MA, Fonarow G, Creaser J, Flavell C, Stevenson LW. Relationship between right and left-sided filling pressures in 1000 patients with advanced heart failure. *J Heart Lung Transplant Off Publ Int Soc Heart Transplant.* 1999;18(11):1126-1132. doi:10.1016/s1053-2498(99)00070-4

188. Drazner MH, Brown RN, Kaiser PA, et al. Relationship of right- and left-sided filling pressures in patients with advanced heart failure: a 14-year multi-institutional analysis. *J Heart Lung Transplant Off Publ Int Soc Heart Transplant.* 2012;31(1):67-72.

doi:10.1016/j.healun.2011.09.003

189. Drazner MH, Prasad A, Ayers C, et al. The relationship of right- and left-sided filling pressures in patients with heart failure and a preserved ejection fraction. *Circ Heart Fail.* 2010;3(2):202-206. doi:10.1161/CIRCHEARTFAILURE.108.876649

190. Campbell P, Drazner MH, Kato M, et al. Mismatch of Right- and Left-Sided Filling Pressures in Chronic Heart Failure. *J Card Fail.* 2011;17(7):561-568. doi:10.1016/j.cardfail.2011.02.013

191. Persistence is omnipotent. Accessed June 29, 2021. https://www.uspto.gov/learning-and-resources/journeys-innovation/field-stories/persistence-omnipotent

192. Halpern SD, Taichman DB. Misclassification of Pulmonary Hypertension Due to Reliance on Pulmonary Capillary Wedge Pressure Rather Than Left Ventricular End-Diastolic Pressure. *Chest.* 2009;136(1):37-43. doi:10.1378/chest.08-2784

193. Hemnes AR, Opotowsky AR, Assad TR, et al. Features Associated With Discordance Between Pulmonary Arterial Wedge Pressure and Left Ventricular End Diastolic Pressure in Clinical Practice: Implications for Pulmonary Hypertension Classification. *Chest.* 2018;154(5):1099-1107. doi:10.1016/j.chest.2018.08.1033

194. Soto FJ, Siegel R, Marks D, et al. Performance of Pulmonary Capillary Wedge Pressure (PCWP) Vs. Left Ventricular End Diastolic Pressure (LVEDP) in the Diagnosis/Classification of Patients with Suspect Pulmonary Arterial Hypertension (PAH). *Chest.* 2005;128(4, Supplement):137S. doi:10.1378/chest.128.4_MeetingAbstracts.137S-a

195. Kafi A, Lindgren B, Chaux G, et al. Low Correlation Between PCWP and LVEDP in Patients With End-Stage Lung Disease. *J Heart Lung Transplant.* 2018;37(4):S450. doi:10.1016/j.healun.2018.01.1170

196. Hansmann G, Rich S, Maron BA. Cardiac catheterization in pulmonary hypertension: doing it right, with a catheter on the left. *Cardiovasc Diagn Ther.* 2020;10(5):1718-1724. doi:10.21037/cdt-20-483

197. Volpicelli G, Skurzak S, Boero E, et al. Lung Ultrasound Predicts Well Extravascular Lung Water but Is of Limited Usefulness in the Prediction of Wedge Pressure. *Anesthesiology.* 2014;121(2):320-327. doi:10.1097/ALN.0000000000000300

198. Agricola E, Picano E, Oppizzi M, et al. Assessment of Stress-induced Pulmonary Interstitial Edema by Chest Ultra-

sound During Exercise Echocardiography and its Correlation with Left Ventricular Function. *J Am Soc Echocardiogr.* 2006;19(4):457-463. doi:10.1016/j.echo.2005.11.013

199. Lichtenstein DA, Mezière GA, Lagoueyte J-F, Biderman P, Goldstein I, Gepner A. A-lines and B-lines: lung ultrasound as a bedside tool for predicting pulmonary artery occlusion pressure in the critically ill. *Chest.* 2009;136(4):1014-1020. doi:10.1378/chest.09-0001

200. Hubert A, Girerd N, Le Breton H, et al. Diagnostic accuracy of lung ultrasound for identification of elevated left ventricular filling pressure. *Int J Cardiol.* 2019;281:62-68. doi:10.1016/j.ijcard.2019.01.055

201. Mandrekar JN. Receiver Operating Characteristic Curve in Diagnostic Test Assessment. *J Thorac Oncol.* 2010;5(9):1315-1316. doi:10.1097/JTO.0b013e3181ec173d

202. Ang S-H, Andrus P. Lung Ultrasound in the Management of Acute Decompensated Heart Failure. *Curr Cardiol Rev.* 2012;8(2):123-136. doi:10.2174/157340312801784907

203. Rivas-Lasarte M, Álvarez-García J, Fernández-Martínez J, et al. Lung ultrasound-guided treatment in ambulatory patients with heart failure: a randomized controlled clinical trial (LUS-HF study). *Eur J Heart Fail.* 2019;21(12):1605-1613. doi:https://doi.org/10.1002/ejhf.1604

204. Araiza-Garaygordobil D, Gopar-Nieto R, Martinez-Amezcua P, et al. A randomized controlled trial of lung ultrasound-guided therapy in heart failure (CLUSTER-HF study). *Am Heart J.* 2020;227:31-39. doi:10.1016/j.ahj.2020.06.003

205. Marini C, Fragasso G, Italia L, et al. Lung ultrasound-guided therapy reduces acute decompensation events in chronic heart failure. *Heart.* 2020;106(24):1934-1939. doi:10.1136/heartjnl-2019-316429

206. Ivens EL, Munt BI. Pericardial disease: what the general cardiologist needs to know. *Heart.* 2007;93(8):993-1000. doi:10.1136/hrt.2005.086587

207. Beck CS. Two Cardiac Compression Triads. *J Am Med Assoc.* 1935;104(9):714-716. doi:10.1001/jama.1935.02760090018005

208. Hanson MG, Chan B. The role of point-of-care ultrasound in the diagnosis of pericardial effusion: a single academic center retrospective study. *Ultrasound J.* 2021;13. doi:10.1186/s13089-021-00205-x

209. Guberman BA, Fowler NO, Engel PJ, Gueron M, Allen JM. Cardiac tamponade in medical patients. *Circulation.* 1981;64(3):633-640. doi:10.1161/01.CIR.64.3.633

210. Gibbs CR, Watson RDS, Singh SP, Lip GYH. Management of pericardial effusion by drainage: a survey of 10 years' experience in a city centre general hospital serving a multiracial population. *Postgrad Med J.* 2000;76(902):809-813. doi:10.1136/pgmj.76.902.809

211. Levine MJ, Lorell BH, Diver DJ, Come PC. Implications of echocardiographically assisted diagnosis of pericardial tamponade in contemporary medical patients: Detection before hemodynamic embarrassment. *J Am Coll Cardiol.* 1991;17(1):59-65. doi:10.1016/0735-1097(91)90704-D

212. Argulian E, Herzog E, Halpern DG, Messerli FH. Paradoxical Hypertension With Cardiac Tamponade. *Am J Cardiol.* 2012;110(7):1066-1069. doi:10.1016/j.amjcard.2012.05.042

213. Brown J, MacKinnon D, King A, Vanderbush E. Elevated Arterial Blood Pressure in Cardiac Tamponade. *N Engl J Med.* 1992;327(7):463-466. doi:10.1056/NEJM199208133270704

214. Cameron E, Istrail L. Diagnosing Early Cardiac Tamponade in Patient with JAK2+ Myeloproliferative Syndrome with Point of Care Ultrasound. *POCUS J.* 2021;6(1):13-15. doi:10.24908/pocus.v6i1.14756

215. Jacob S, Sebastian JC, Cherian PK, Abraham A, John SK. Pericardial effusion impending tamponade: a look beyond Beck's triad. *Am J Emerg Med.* 2009;27(2):216-219. doi:10.1016/j.ajem.2008.01.056

216. Roy CL, Minor MA, Brookhart MA, Choudhry NK. Does This Patient With a Pericardial Effusion Have Cardiac Tamponade? *JAMA.* 2007;297(16):1810. doi:10.1001/jama.297.16.1810

217. Curtiss EI, Reddy PS, Uretsky BF, Cecchetti AA. Pulsus paradoxus: definition and relation to the severity of cardiac tamponade. *Am Heart J.* 1988;115(2):391-398. doi:10.1016/0002-8703(88)90487-5

218. Singh S, Wann LS, Klopfenstein HS, Hartz A, Brooks HL. Usefulness of right ventricular diastolic collapse in diagnosing cardiac tamponade and comparison to pulsus paradoxus. *Am J Cardiol.* 1986;57(8):652-656. doi:10.1016/0002-9149(86)90853-2

219. Argulian E, Messerli F. Misconceptions and facts about pericardial effusion and tamponade. *Am J Med.* 2013;126(10):858-861. doi:10.1016/j.amjmed.2013.03.022

220. Van Dam MN, Fitzgerald BM. Pulsus Paradoxus. In: *Stat-Pearls*. StatPearls Publishing; 2021. Accessed September 4, 2021. http://www.ncbi.nlm.nih.gov/books/NBK482292/

221. Textbook of Clinical Echocardiography. Accessed July 2, 2021. https://www.us.elsevierhealth.com/textbook-of-clinical-echocardiography-9780323480482.html

222. Himelman RB, Kircher B, Rockey DC, Schiller NB. Inferior vena cava plethora with blunted respiratory response: A sensitive echocardiography sign of cardiac tamponade. *J Am Coll Cardiol*. 1988;12(6):1470-1477. doi:10.1016/S0735-1097(88)80011-1

223. Stone MB, Huang JV. Inferior Vena Cava Assessment: Correlation with CVP and Plethora in Tamponade. *Glob Heart*. 2013;8(4):323-327. doi:10.1016/j.gheart.2013.11.004

224. UltrasoundPod. *Ultrasound Podcast - PERICARDIAL TAMPONADE. LEARN THIS. KNOW THIS*. Accessed July 3, 2021. https://www.youtube.com/watch?v=s-qwWg_AlD0&t=1076s

225. Alpert EA, Amit U, Guranda L, Mahagna R, Grossman SA, Bentancur A. Emergency department point-of-care ultrasonography improves time to pericardiocentesis for clinically significant effusions. *Clin Exp Emerg Med*. 2017;4(3):128-132. doi:10.15441/ceem.16.169

226. Get A Horse! America's Skepticism Toward the First Automobiles. The Saturday Evening Post. Published January 9, 2017. Accessed July 7, 2021. https://www.saturdayeveningpost.com/2017/01/get-horse-americas-skepticism-toward-first-automobiles/

227. The Horseless Age: A monthly Journal. Accessed July 12, 2021. http://www.carsandracingstuff.com/library/h/horselessage1896b.pdf

228. Corcoran JP, Laursen CB. COUNTERPOINT: Should Point-of-Care Ultrasound Examination Be Routine Practice in the Evaluation of the Acutely Breathless Patient? No. *CHEST*. 2019;156(3):426-428. doi:10.1016/j.chest.2019.04.119

229. Koenig S, Tsegaye A. Rebuttal From Drs Koenig and Tsegaye. *Chest*. 2019;156(3):428-429. doi:10.1016/j.chest.2019.04.116

230. Copetti R, Vetrugno L, Orso D, Bove T. Should the Stethoscope Auscultation Be Routine Practice in the Evaluation of the Acutely Breathless Patient? No. *Chest*. 2020;157(3):740-742. doi:10.1016/j.chest.2019.09.043

231. Bernstein L. Heart doctors are listening for clues to the future of their stethoscopes. *Washington Post*. https://www.washing-

tonpost.com/national/health-science/heart-doctors-are-listen-ing-for-clues-to-the-future-of-their-stethoscopes/2016/01/02/bd73b000-a98d-11e5-8058-480b572b4aae_story.html. Pub-lished January 2, 2016. Accessed August 12, 2021.

232. First Ultrasound-on- a-Chip receives broadest FDA 510(k) clearance | Butterfly iQ+. Accessed September 14, 2021. https://www.butterflynetwork.com/press-releases/first-ultrasound-on-a-chip-receives-broadest-fda-510-k-clearance

233. Fred HL. Hyposkillia. *Tex Heart Inst J*. 2005;32(3):255-257.

234. The Great Influenza by John M. Barry: 9780143036494 | PenguinRandomHouse.com: Books. Penguin-Randomhouse.com. Accessed July 16, 2021. https://www.pen-guinrandomhouse.com/books/288950/the-great-influenza-by-john-m-barry/

235. Roelandt JRTC. Ultrasound stethoscopy: a renaissance of the physical examination? *Heart*. 2003;89(9):971-973. doi:10.1136/heart.89.9.971

236. Bernstein E, Wang TY. Point-of-Care Ultrasonography: Visually Satisfying Medicine or Evidence-Based Medicine? *JAMA Intern Med*. Published online October 11, 2021. doi:10.1001/jamain-ternmed.2021.5831

237. Koenig SJ, Lou BX, Moskowitz Y, Narasimhan M, Mayo PH. Ultrasound Billing for Intensivists. *Chest*. 2019;156(4):792-801. doi:10.1016/j.chest.2019.06.006

238. Soni NJ, Schnobrich D, Mathews BK, et al. Point-of-Care Ultra-sound for Hospitalists: A Position Statement of the Society of Hospital Medicine. *J Hosp Med*. 2019;14:E1-E6. doi:10.12788/jhm.3079

239. Istrail. Is It Time to Ditch the Stethoscope? Doximity. Accessed July 12, 2021. https://www.doximity.com/newsfeed/4f18f633-b1b9-480b-ba4a-f0411430b43f

240. Andersen CA, Brodersen J, Rudbæk TR, Jensen MB. Patients' ex-periences of the use of point-of-care ultrasound in general prac-tice – a cross-sectional study. *BMC Fam Pract*. 2021;22(1):116. doi:10.1186/s12875-021-01459-z

241. Dversdal M.D., Renee. On POCUS in your practice. Published on-line July 9, 2021.

242. Soni M.D., N. Interview with Nilam Soni. Published online Au-gust 5, 2021.

243. Koratala MD A. POCUS in nephrology. Published online August 4, 2021.

244. Wiskar M.D. K. Interview with Dr. Katie Wiskar. Published online August 10, 2021.

245. Butterfly Network. *Anesthesiology Ultrasound: Dr. Jonny Wilkinson.* Accessed August 17, 2021. https://www.youtube.com/watch?v=zSJzQP9OvJA

246. Wilkinson DrJ. POCUS in the ICU. Published online August 16, 2021.

247. Butterfly Network. *Medical Education: UC Irvine White Coat Ceremony 2019.* Accessed August 10, 2021. https://www.youtube.com/watch?v=fmGZ84KkF3A

248. Nevada TU. Touro University Nevada Partners with Vave Health to Bring Portable Ultrasounds to College of Osteopathic Medical Students - Touro Nevada. Accessed August 21, 2021. https://tun.touro.edu/about-us/news/2020/october/touro-university-nevada-partners-with-vave-health-to-bring-portable-ultrasounds-to-college-of-osteopathic-medical-students.php

249. Lewis Katz School of Medicine is the First Medical School in Philadelphia and the East Coast to Provide All First-Year Students with Butterfly iQ+ Ultrasound Devices | Lewis Katz School of Medicine at Temple University. Accessed August 21, 2021. https://medicine.temple.edu/news/lewis-katz-school-medicine-first-medical-school-philadelphia-and-east-coast-provide-all-first

250. Lewis Katz School of Medicine at Temple University. *Class of 2025 - Butterfly Ultrasound Devices Reveal.* Accessed August 21, 2021. https://www.youtube.com/watch?v=kMJN_xKWp6M

251. Fox M.D. C. Zoom Interview with Dr. Fox. Published online August 4, 2021.

252. POCUS Certificate of Completion. Accessed August 14, 2021. https://www.hospitalmedicine.org/clinical-topics/ultrasound/pocus-certificate-of-completion/

253. The Empath (episode). Memory Alpha. Accessed August 14, 2021. https://memory-alpha.fandom.com/wiki/The_Empath_(episode)

254. NMTVideos. *Star Trek Medical Scanner.* Accessed August 14, 2021. https://www.youtube.com/watch?v=IHd9bYGJtoI

255. -scope | Origin and meaning of suffix -scope by Online Etymology Dictionary. Accessed July 18, 2021. https://www.etymonline.com/word/-scope

256. Barach JH. Stethophone, Not Stethoscope. *J*

Am Med Assoc. 1913;61(25):2260-2260. doi:10.1001/jama.1913.04350260058026

257. Our Mission - Butterfly Network. Accessed August 15, 2021. https://www.butterflynetwork.com/our-mission

258. Vave Health Home. Vave Health. Accessed August 15, 2021. https://vavehealth.com/

259. Portable Pocket Handheld Ultrasound Scanners - Clarius. Clarius Mobile Health. Accessed August 15, 2021. https://clarius.com/

260. Sonosite PX | Sonosite. Accessed August 15, 2021. https://www.sonosite.com/products/sonosite-px

261. Venous Thrombosis during Spaceflight | NEJM. Accessed August 15, 2021. https://www.nejm.org/doi/full/10.1056/NEJMc1905875

262. FAST at MACH 20: Clinical Ultrasound Aboard the Internationa...: Journal of Trauma and Acute Care Surgery. Accessed August 15, 2021. https://journals.lww.com/jtrauma/Fulltext/2005/01000/Focused_Assessment_with_Sonography_for_Trauma.00006.aspx?casa_token=k-unSqzNwCEAAAAA:dlyY-iItw4wjigOBv5LSZI2N6hq3GcZEjSlDlJfvZuS5KCnfipop-KaVB4yBthSvAMahELUoTKTFDRUT2F20olRFTG

263. Inspiration4 Mission. Baylor College of Medicine. Accessed September 30, 2021. https://www.bcm.edu/academic-centers/space-medicine/translational-research-institute/research/inspiration4-mission

264. Jr DGM, Mbabazi ER. In African Villages, These Phones Become Ultrasound Scanners. *The New York Times.* https://www.nytimes.com/2019/04/15/health/medical-scans-butterfly-iq.html. Published April 15, 2019. Accessed August 15, 2021.

---

[1] The disease Laennec himself would succumb to 40 years later, diagnosed with the device he invented and the field of diagnostic medicine he pioneered.

[2] In the ultimate morbid tribute, this technique would eventually be used to diagnose Laennec himself with tuberculosis, shortly before his death.

[3] Lichtenstein prides himself on rarely ordering a CT scan unless absolutely necessary. He felt that using a CT scan for research exposed patients to unnecessary radiation and he was very opposed to this. Almost all of the CT scans he compared his work to had been ordered by other clinicians.

[4] Many of the PAH drugs we use today were developed by Martine Rothblatt, the founder of Sirius Satellite Radio. In a miraculous story, she led the de-

velopment of a whole new drug pipeline for pulmonary hypertension in an attempt to save her daughter's life, ultimately starting *United Therapeutics*, where her daughter now works.[191]

Made in the USA
Las Vegas, NV
02 September 2022